i10 Cheat Sheet
for Home Health

Diagnostic Codes for Adult Patients

Simplify your coding!
Speedify your coding!

FY 2016

GLB Worldwide . Jerry Gill

i10 Cheat Sheet for Home Health © Copyright 2015 Jerry Gill

Published by GLB Worldwide *"Great Little Books"*
POBox 6495   Kaneohe HI 96744

ISBN 13   978 1516948123

ISBN 10   1516948122

Find it on Amazon and on the following web sites

http://www.icd10cheatsheet.com

http://www.glbworld.com

If you have time, a review on Amazon is always appreciated.

If you have suggestions, send them
info@glbworld.com

Using The Cheat Sheet

The i10 Cheat Sheet for Home Health has one goal - to make coding faster and less hassle for those who work in home care and tend to already have a daunting 'to do' list. Since it is a cheat sheet it obviously doesn't have all codes but does include *thousands* of codes repeatedly used in home health care.

Common diagnosis acronyms have been coded as in the icd-9 Cheat Sheet. Some of those are OB, pedi or neo. Other than those acronyms, all codes in the i10 Cheat Sheet are for non-traumatic diagnosis codes for non-OB adult patients.

If you used the icd-9 Cheat Sheet, you will find the i10 version similar and as easy to use. There are some differences, though. The breadth of the icd-9 version has been joined by more depth.

Many entries will display 'RELATED' codes which may or may not be useful. They are conditions that often accompany the main term of an entry. If you don't need the related code, ignore it. If you need it, that's one less lookup.

Neoplasm entries show 'METS' codes. These serve the same purpose as 'related' codes. They are codes for secondary neoplasms that may occur with the main entry — another time you may need one less lookup.

For most entries there is a code to the left of the title entry. That code is for that title entry as written. Codes for similar varieties, types, locations, etc. may be listed below it and will be accompanied by their appropriate descriptions.
For example: if you are looking up a code for a leg or arm condition, the main entry is likely the condition for 'unspecified' or NOS. Below will be listed the codes for specified right, left, and bilateral.

The Cheat Sheet is set up alphabetically by anatomy - mostly. If a diagnosis is usually or always associated with a site, that is how it is listed. Pressure ulcer of the buttock and gout of the toe will be found at buttock and toe. If site / location is unnecessary to describe a diagnosis, the diagnosis is listed under the generally used term, usually the common name. Lobar pneumonia and alcoholic ataxia are found at pneumonia and ataxia. If you don't find the code you need at a site, it may be listed at the higher level anatomical site. For example, to code an abscess of the thigh, look at leg abscess. Occasionally terms have two locations. Osteoporosis with a shoulder fracture will be found at shoulder. At Osteoporosis you will find general codes to use if there is no current fracture.

USING THE CHEAT SHEET: The most often used strategy is to go through all your coding with the Cheat Sheet first. If you have several patients to code, go through them all with the Cheat Sheet. Many patients can be completed with the Cheat Sheet alone. If any diagnosis could not be coded with the Cheat Sheet, go to a complete reference. Using this method can lessen considerably the time you spend coding. The official pdf version of diagnostic codes from CMS can be downloaded free at http://www.icd10cheatsheet.com.

The Cheat Sheet has ample margins for making your own notations. If you find codes not in the Cheat Sheet but which you use frequently in your patient population, add them on the page they would be listed. If you add notations to your Cheat Sheet, it would be greatly appreciated if you'd let us know. They will be included in the next edition. Just send them to info@glbworld.com.

Abbreviations you'll encounter
unsp unspec - unspecified
NOS - not otherwise specified
NEC - not elsewhere classified / coded
w/ with   w/o without
/ or   d//t due to

Consider the terms 'NOS' and 'unspecified' as equal and are used when diagnosis information is incomplete.

"Other" codes are used for a condition that has a description but no matching code.

A dash at the end or within a sequence of code characters indicates that you need to insert a character and choices are provided.

i10 Cheat Sheet for Home Care

I714	**AAA: aortic abdominal aneurysm w/o rupture**
	w/rupture I713
R100	**Abdomen acute**
K660	**Abdomen adhesions postinfection / postop NOS**
	postinfection / postop w/obstruction K565
M79A3	**Abdomen compartment syndrome nontraumatic**
I714	**Abdominal aneurysm aorta**
	w/ rupture I713
K551	**Abdominal angina**
T79A3X-	**Abdominal compartment syndrome traumatic**
	7th character indicates encounter (trauma only) -
	A - initial encounter D - subsequent encounter S - sequela
	nontraumatic M79A3
R109	**Abdominal cramps NOS**
R140	**Abdominal distension**
K632	**Abdominal fistula (wall)**
R188	**Abdominal fluid accumulation NOS**
K469	**Abdominal hernia NOS**
	w/gangrene K461 w/obstruction K460
	ventral incisional/postop NOS K432 w/gangrene K431
	ventral NOS K439
R1084	**Abdominal pain generalized NOS**
R1030	**Abdominal pain local lower NOS**
	RLQ R1031 LLQ R1032
	periumbilical R1033
R1010	**Abdominal pain local upper NOS**
	RUQ R1011 LUQ R1012
	epigastric R1013
R1930	**Abdominal rigidity NOS**
	RUQ R1931 LUQ R1932
	RLQ R1933 LLQ R1934
	periumbilic R1935 epigastric R1936
	generalized R1937
R1900	**Abdominal swelling, mass, lump NOS**
	RUQ R1901 LUQ R1902
	RLQ R1903 LLQ R1904
	Periumbilic R1905 Epigastric R1906
	Generalized R1907 Other R1909
R10819	**Abdominal tenderness NOS**
	RUQ R10811 LUQ R10812
	RLQ R10813 LLQ R10814
	periumbilic R10815 epigastric R10816
	generalized R10817

R10829	**Abdominal tenderness REBOUND NOS**
	RUQ R10821 LUQ R10822
	RLQ R10823 LLQ R10824
	periumbilic R10825 epigastric R10826
	generalized R10827
L02211	**Abdominal wall abscess cutaneous, code organism if known**
L02231	**Abdominal wall carbuncle, code organism if known**
K632	**Abdominal wall fistula NOS**
L02221	**Abdominal wall furuncle/boil, code organism if known**
I330	**ABE: acute bacterial endocarditis**
L0390	**Abscess NOS**
-	**Abuse of non-psychoactive substances**
	antacids F550 herbal / folk remedies F551
	laxative F552 steroids / hormones F553
	vitamins F554 other F558
B889	**Acariasis NOS**
K900	**ACD: adult celiac disease**
R824	**Acetonuria**
K220	**Achalasia NOS / cardia / esophageal**
M7660	**Achilles tendinitis unsp**
	right M7661 left M7662
K3183	**Achlorhydria**
E872	**Acidosis lactic/metabolic/NOS/propionic/respiratory**
	renal / kidney tubular N2589
G803	**ACP: athetoid cerebral palsy**
-	**Acromioclavicular joint dislocation**
	unsp S43109- right S43101- left S43102-
	7th character indicates encounter
	A - initial encounter D - subsequent encounter S - sequela
-	**Acromioclavicular sprain**
	unsp S4350x- right S4361x- left S4362x-
	7th character indicates encounter
	A - initial encounter D - subsequent encounter S - sequela
M5382	**ACS: acute cervical spine syndrome**
A429	**Actinomycosis NOS**
	Pulmonary A420 sepsis A427
	Abdominal A421
	Cervicofacial A422
	meningitis A42.81 encephalitis A4282
	Other forms A4289
	RELATED cystitis N3080 w/ hematuria N3081
	RELATED meningitis G01
	RELATED prostatis N51
F909	**ADD: attention deficit disorder NOS**
	predominantly inattentive F900
	predominantly hyperactive F901
	combined type F902
	other F908

E271	**Addison's disease primary (adrenocortical insufficiency)**
	crisis E272 NOS E2740 drug induced E273
	tuberculous A187
	RELATED Addison's anemia D510
G0400	**ADEM: acute disseminated encephalitis and encephalomyelitis NOS**
	postinfectious G0401
	postimmunization G0402
	noninfectious G0481
-	**Adenitis - SEE Lymphadenitis**
J358	**Adenoid vegetations**
J3503	**Adenoiditis & tonsillitis chronic**
	adenoiditis alone chronic J3502
-	**ADHD: attention deficit hyperactivity disorder SEE ADD**
E342	**ADHES: antidiuretic hormone secretion ectopic (ADH)**
E222	**ADHIS: antidiuretic hormone secretion inappropriate (SIADH)**
T50905-	**ADR: adverse drug reaction, unspecified drug**
	penicillins T360x5- tetracyclines T365x5-
	sulfonamide T370x5- insulin & oral antidiabetics T383x5-
	aspirin T39015- other salicylates T39095-
	other NSAIDS T39395- barbiturates T423x5-
	antiallergic / antiemetic T450x5- antineoplastic T451x5-
	anticoagulant T45515- antithrombotic T45525-
	thrombolytic T45615- hemostatic T45625-
	coronary vasodilator T463x5- antivaricose T468x5-
	7th character indicates encounter
	A - initial encounter D - subsequent encounter S - sequela
-	**Adrenal hyperplasia SEE Cushing's Syndrome**
E259	**Adrenogenital syndrome NOS**
T50905-	**Adverse effect, unspecified drug**
	penicillins T360x5- tetracyclines T365x5-
	sulfonamide T370x5- insulin & oral antidiabetics T383x5-
	aspirin T39015- other salicylates T39095-
	other NSAIDS T39395- barbiturates T423x5-
	antiallergic / antiemetic T450x5- antineoplastic T451x5-
	anticoagulant T45515- antithrombotic T45525-
	thrombolytic T45615- hemostatic T45625-
	coronary vasodilator T463x5- antivaricose T468x5-
	7th character indicates encounter
	A - initial encounter D - subsequent encounter S - sequela
Z7901	**Aftercare anticoagulant use long term current**
	RELATED drug level monitoring Z5181
Z483	**Aftercare following surgery for neoplasm**
Z5189	**Aftercare NOS SEE specific type also, eg wound, colostomy**
	NEC Z5189
	postop orthopedic joint replacement Z471
	postop drain: change Z4803 removal Z4889
	tracheostomy Z430

-	**Aftercare orthopedic**
	Z471 following joint replacement surgery
	Z472 for removal of internal fixation device
	Z4733 following explantation of knee joint prosthesis
	Z4732 following explantation of hip joint prosthesis
	Z4731 following explantation of shoulder joint prosthesis
	Z4782 following scoliosis surgery
	Z4781 following surgical amputation
	Use additional code to identify limb amputated (Z89.-)
	Z4789 other orthopedic aftercare
Z48815	**Aftercare postop digestive system**
N009	**AGN: acute glomerulonephritis**
D66	**AHGD: antihemophilic globulin deficiency**
T80310-	**AHTR: acute hemolytic transfusion reaction d/t ABO incompatibility within 24 hrs of transfusion**
	d/t Rh incompatibility T80410-
	7th character indicates encounter
	A - initial encounter D - subsequent encounter S - sequela
-	**AICD complication**
	mechanical breakdown T82518-
	displacement T82528-
	leakage T82538-
	Infection T827xx-
	7th character indicates encounter
	A - initial encounter D - subsequent encounter S - sequela
Z4502	**AICD defibrillator fitting & adjustment**
Z95810	**AICD status**
Z717	**Aids counseling**
R75	**Aids HIV lab evidence inconclusive**
Z21	**Aids infection asymptomatic status / HIV positive**
B20	**AIDS: acquired immunodeficiency syndrome**
	RELATED Kaposi's sarcomas:
	gastrointestinal organ C464
	palate (hard) (soft) C462
	rectum C464 lymph node(s) C463
	lung: unsp C4650 right C4651 left C4652
	Kaposi's varicelliform eruption B000
K6282	**AIN: anal intraepithelial neoplasia (histologically confirmed) NOS/grade I /grade II**
	grade III, severe D013
E8021	**AIP: acute intermittent porphyria**
T800XX-	**Air embolism following infusion, transfusion and therapeutic injection**
	7th character indicates encounter
	A - initial encounter D - subsequent encounter S - sequela
N179	**AKF: acute kidney failure NOS nontraumatic**
	w/tubular necrosis N170
	w/acute cortical necrosis N171
	w/medullary necrosis N172
	other spec N178

F1010	**Alcohol abuse uncomplicated**
	w/intoxication: uncomplicated F10120 delirium F10121 unsp F10129
	alcohol induced psychosis w/ delusions F10150
	alcoholhallucinations F10151 unsp F10159
	alcohol induced: anxiety F10180 sexual dysfunction F10181
	alcohol induced: sleep disorder F10182 other disorder F10188
	alcohol induced mood disorder F1014
	abuse w/unsp disorder F1019
F10231	**Alcohol withdrawal delirium**
F10239	**Alcohol withdrawal syndrome/psychosis NOS**
Z6372	**Alcoholism in family**
F1020	**Alcoholism NOS**
	in remission F1021
	w/mood disorder F1024
	w/persisting dementia F1027
E269	**Aldosteronism NOS (also hyperaldosteronism)**
	other primary E2609 Secondary E261
	Bartler's E2681
	Conn's syndrome E2601
	glucocorticoid-remediable E2602
R29898	**ALF: acute loss of function**
E873	**Alkalosis NOS**
C9100	**ALL: acute lymphoid leukemia NOS**
	in remission C9101 in relapse C9102
Z880	**Allergy to penicillin**
Z91013	**Allergy to seafood**
G3181	**Alpers disease**
D8982	**ALPS: autoimmune lymphoproliferative syndrome**
G1221	**ALS: amyotrophic lateral sclerosis**
G309	**Alzheimer's disease NOS**
	early onset G300 late onset G301
	other G308
	RELATED dementia w/behavioral disturbance F0281
	RELATED dementia w/o behavioral disturbance F0280
	RELATED delerium F05
-	**Ambulation difficulty SEE WALKING**
-	**AMD: age related macular degenertion SEE ARMD**
A069	**Amebiasis**
	acute dysentery A060 chronic intestinal A061
	nondysenteric colitis A062 Ameboma A063
	hepatic A064 brain abscess A066
	cystitis A0681
I213	**AMI: acute myocardial infarction NOS**
A319	**AMI: atypical mycobacterial infection NOS**
	cutaneous A311 pulmonary A310
C9200	**AML: acute myeloid leukemia NOS**
	in remission C9201 in relapse C9202
R413	**Amnesia NOS**
	anterograde R411 retrograde R412

E859	**Amyloidosis unsp**
	non-neuropathic E850
	neuropathic E851
	heredofamilial E852
	secondary systemic / hemodialysis associated E853
	localized E854
	other E858
E3450	**Androgen sensitivity syndrome NOS**
	complete E3451 partial E3452
D519	**Anemia B12 deficiency NOS**
	d/t intrinsic factor deficiency D510
	d/t selective malabsorption D511
	other dietary deficiency D513
	other D518
	transcobalamin II deficiency D512
D529	**Anemia folate deficiency NOS**
	dietary deficiency D520
	drug-induced D521
	other D528
D599	**Anemia hemolytic acquired NOS**
	autoimmune: drug induced D590 other D591
	nonautoimmune: drug induced D592 other D594
	hemolytic-uremic syndrom D593
	other D598
D509	**Anemia iron deficiency NOS**
	secondary to blood loss D500
	secondary to inadequate intake D508
	sideropenic dysphagia D501
D539	**Anemia nutritional NOS / simple chronic**
	scorbutic D532
	protein D530
	other nutritional D538
	megaloblastic NOS D531
D62	**Anemia posthemorrhagic acute**
	d/t chronic blood loss D500
D530	**Anemia protein deficiency**
D513	**Anemia vegan**
I209	**Angina pectoris NOS**
	unstable I200
	w/documented spasm I201 other I208
	postinfarction I237
	RELATED exp to environmental smoke NOS Z7722
	RELATED exp to environmental smoke occupational Z5731
	RELATED hx of tobacco use Z87891 tobacco use Z720
G0430	**ANHE: acute necrotizing hemorrhagic encephalopathy NOS**
	postinfectious G0431
	postimmunization G0432
	other G0439

L02429	**Ankle boil / furuncle unspecified**
	right L02425 left L02426
	Unspecified code is good for any "limb"
M71479	**Ankle calcification unsp**
	right M71471 left M71472
L02439	**Ankle carbuncle unsp side**
	right L02435 left L02436
	Unspecified code is good for any "limb"
M9279	**Ankle chondromalacia unsp**
	right M94271 left M94272
M24573	**Ankle contractures unsp**
	right M24571 left M24572
M25473	**Ankle effusion unsp**
	right M25471 left M25472
-	**Ankle fracture pathological NOS / in neoplastic disease**
	unsp M84473- right M84471- left M84472-
	7th character indicates encounter/status
	A - initial S - sequela
	D - subsequent routine healing
	G - subsequent delayed healing
	K - subsequent nonunion P - subsequent malunion
	Change 4th character to 5 for 'in neoplastic disease'
M25073	**Ankle hemarthrosis unsp**
	right M25071 left M25072
M24873	**Ankle instability NOS unsp**
	right M24871 left M24872
M24073	**Ankle joint mice unsp**
	right M24071 left M24072
-	**Ankle osteomyelitis**
	acute hematogenous: unsp M86079 right M86071 left M86072
	other acute: unsp M86179 right M86171 left M86172
	subacute: unsp M86279 right M86271 left M86272
	chronic multifocal: unsp M86379 right M86371 left M86372
	chronic, draining sinus: unsp M86479 right M86471 left 86472
	chronic hematogenous: unsp M86579 right M86571 left M86572
	other chronic: unsp M86679 right M86671 left M86672
M80079-	**Ankle osteoporosis age related w/current fracture unsp**
	right M80071- left M80072-
	7th character indicates encounter/status
	A - initial D - subsequent routine healing
	G - subsequent delayed healing S - sequela
	K - subsequent nonunion P - subsequent malunion
L89529	**Ankle pressure ulcer left NOS**
	unstageable L89520
	stage 1 L89521 stage 2 L89522
	stage 3 L89523 stage 4 L89524

L89519	**Ankle pressure ulcer right NOS**
	unstageable L89510
	stage 1 L89511 stage 2 L89512
	stage 3 L89513 stage 4 L89514
L89509	**Ankle pressure ulcer unspecified side NOS**
	unstageable L89500
	stage 1 L89501 stage 2 L89502
	stage 3 L89503 stage 4 L89504
M25673	**Ankle stiffness (joint) NOS unsp**
	right M25671 left M25672
-	**Ankle swelling (joint) SEE ankle effusion**
L97329	**Ankle ulcer non-pressure chronic left NOS**
	limited to skin L97321
	w/fat layer exposed L97322
	w/muscle necrosis L97323
	w/bone necrosis L97324
L97319	**Ankle ulcer non-pressure chronic right NOS**
	limited to skin L97311
	w/fat layer exposed L97312
	w/muscle necrosis L97313
	w/bone necrosis L97314
L97309	**Ankle ulcer non-pressure chronic unspecified side NOS**
	limited to skin L97301
	w/fat layer exposed L97302
	w/muscle necrosis L97303
	w/bone necrosis L97304
-	**Anogenital herpes SEE Herpes simplex Anogenital**
K612	**Anorectal abscess / cellulitis**
K605	**Anorectal fistula**
F5000	**Anorexia nervosa NOS**
	restricting type F5001
	binge eating/purging type F5002
R630	**Anorexia NOS (simple, loss of appetite)**
K859	**ANP: acute necrotizing pancreatitis**
I808	**Antecubital thrombophlebitis**
G8382	**Anterior cord syndrome**
D6832	**Anticoagulant induced hemorrhage**
Z7901	**Anticoagulant use long term current - includes aftercare**
	RELATED drug level monitoring Z5181
A691	**ANUG: acute necrotizing ulcerative gingivitis**
R34	**Anuria NOS**
	postop N990
	traumatic T795XX-
	for traumatic code 7th character indicates encounter
	A - initial encounter D - subsequent encounter S - sequela
K610	**Anus abscess / cellulitis**
K6289	**Anus cyst NOS**
K6282	**Anus dysplasia NOS**

K602	**Anus fissure NOS**

        acute K600   chronic K601

K603	**Anus fistula**
K6289	**Anus granuloma/ irritation NOS**
K625	**Anus hemorrhage**
A563	**Anus infection d/t chlamydia trachomatis**
-	**Anus neoplasm**

        malignant unsp C210
        malignant canal   C211
        malignant cloacogenic zone   C212
        malignant overlapping sites w/rectum C218
        Secondary   C785
        Benign D129
        Mets to bone   C7951   mets to unsp lymph nodes C779
        Mets to intraabdominal lymph node C772
        Mets to intrapelvic lymph node C775

K620	**Anus polyp**
K622	**Anus prolapse**
K624	**Anus stenosis/stricture**
A1832	**Anus tuberculosis NOS**
F419	**Anxiety NOS**
I719	**Aorta aneurysm NOS**

        NOS w/rupture I718
        thoracic: NOS I712 ruptured I711
        abdominal: NOS I714   ruptured I713
        thoracoabdominal: NOS I716 ruptured I715

I700	**Aorta atherosclerosis NOS**
I7100	**Aorta dissection NOS**

        thoracic I7101   abdominal I7102
        thoracoabdominal I7103

I7410	**Aorta embolism and thrombosis NOS**

        abdominal saddle embolus I7401
        abdominal other I7409
        thoracic I7411   other I7419

I359	**Aortic valve disorder nonrheumatic unsp**

        stenosis I350   insufficiency I351
        stenosis w/insufficiency I352
        other I358

T8201XA	**Aortic valve prosthesis mechanical malfunction initial encounter**

        subsequent encounter T8201XD
        sequela T8201XS

I351	**Aortic valve regurgitation NOS**

        rheumatic I061

I062	**Aortic valve rheumatic stenosis w/insufficiency**

        stenosis NOS I060

J810	**APE: acute pulmonary edema**
I2699	**APE: acute pulmonary embolism NOS**
R130	**Aphagia NOS**

        psychogenic F509

R4701	**Aphasia ataxic/ Broca's/ expressive/ motor/ NOS/ sensory**
	specified as sequelae of CVA or CVD late effect I69920
Q612	**APKD: adult type polycystic kidney disease congenital**
C9240	**APL: acute promyelocytic leukemia NOS**
	in remission C9241 in relapse C9242
-	**Apnea Sleep - SEE sleep apnea**
G039	**Arachnoiditis spinal NOS**
B20	**ARC: aids related complex**
J80	**ARDS: acute respiratory distress syndrome**
N179	**ARF: acute renal failure NOS**
	w/ acute cortical necrosis N171
	w/ medullary necrosis N172
	w/ tubular n N170
L02413	**Arm abscess cutaneous right, code organism if known**
	left L02414
I721	**Arm artery aneurysm**
-	**Arm bone cyst**
	solitary humerus: unsp M85429 right M85421 left M85422
	solitary forearm: unsp M85439 right M85431 left M85432
	aneurysmal cyst: change 4th digit to 5
	other cyst: change 4th digit to 6
L02433	**Arm carbuncle right, code organism if known**
	left L02434
G5640	**Arm causalgia NOS**
	right G5641 left G5642
-	**Arm compartment syndrome**
	nontraumatic: right M79A11 left M79A12 unsp M79A19
	traumatic: right T79A11- left T79A12- unsp T79A19-
	For traumatic codes, 7th character indicates encounter
	A - initial encounter D - subsequent encounter S - sequela
	Includes all sites from shoulder to fingers
I82629	**Arm deep vein thrombosis acute NOS**
	right I82621 left I82622 bilateral I82623
I82729	**Arm deep vein thrombosis chronic NOS**
	right I82721 left I82722 bilateral I82723
	personal history of deep vein thrombosis Z86718
R600	**Arm edema pitting/dependent/NOS**
-	**Arm embolism/thrombosis venous**
	deep: acute I82629 chronic I82729
	superficial: acute I82619 chronic I82719
	NOS: acute I82609 chronic I82709

-	**Arm fracture pathological NOS / in neoplastic disease**
	humerus: unsp M84429- right M84421- left M84422-
	ulna: right M84431- left M84432-
	radius: right M84433- left M84434-
	forearm: unsp M84439-
	7th character indicates encounter/status
	A - initial S - sequela
	D - subsequent routine healing
	G - subsequent delayed healing
	K - subsequent nonunion P - subsequent malunion
	Change 4th character to 5 for 'in neoplastic disease'
L02423	**Arm furuncle/boil right**
	left L02424
R2230	**Arm lump/mass/swelling skin NOS**
	right R2231 left R2232 bilat R2233
G5690	**Arm mononeuropathy NOS**
	right G5691 left G5692
G8320	**Arm monoplegia NOS**
	dominant side: right G8321 left G8322
	nondominant: right G8323 left G8324
-	**Arm osteonecrosis 4th character below**
	humerus: unsp M87-29 right M87-21 left M87-22
	radius: unsp M87-33 right M87-31 left M87-32
	ulna: unsp M87-36 right M87-34 left M87-35
	shoulder: unsp M87-19 right M87-11 left M87-12
	carpus: unsp M87-39 right M87-37 left M87-38
	hand: unsp M87-43 right M87-41 left M87-42
	finger: unsp M87-46 right M87-44 left M87-45
	4th character
	idiopathic aseptic = 0 d/t drugs = 1 d/t trauma = 2
	other secondary = 3 other = 8
-	**Arm osteoporosis age related w/current pathological fracture**
	shoulder: unsp M80019- right M80011- left M80012-
	humerus: unsp M80029- right M80021- left M80022-
	forearm: unsp M80039- right M80031- left M80032-
	hand: unsp M80049- right M80041- left M80042-
	7th character indicates encounter/status
	A - initial S - sequela
	D - subsequent routine healing
	G - subsequent delayed healing
	K - subsequent nonunion P - subsequent malunion
I742	**Arm peripheral disease occlusive**
H3530	**ARMD: age related macular degeneration NOS (also AMD)**
	exudative H3532 non-exudative H3531
I770	**Arteriovenous fistula acquired**
T82390-	**Arteriovenous shunt clot/malfunction/mechanical failure**
	infected T827XX-
	7th character indicates encounter
	A - initial encounter D - subsequent encounter S - sequela

T827XX-	**Arteriovenous shunt infected**	
	7th character indicates encounter	
	A - initial encounter D - subsequent encounter S - sequela	
-	**Artery disorders**	
	septic embolism I76	
	arteriovenous fistula I770	
	narrowing / stricture I771 rupture / ulcer I772	
	fibromuscular dysplasia I773	
	necrosis I775 arteritis NOS I776	
	unspecified I779	
I7779	**Artery dissection NOS other**	
	carotid I7771 iliac I7772	
	renal I7773 vertebral I7774	
M2550	**Arthralgia NOS**	
	shoulder: right M25511 left M25512 unsp M25519	
	elbow: right M25521 left M25522 unsp M25529	
	wrist: right M25531 left M25532 unsp M25539	
	hip: right M25551 left M25552 unsp M25559	
	knee: right M25561 left M25562 unsp M25569	
	ankle & foot: M25571 right left M25572 unsp M25579	
M129	**Arthritis NOS**	
R87611	**ASC-H: atypical squamous cells cannot exclude high grade squamous intrepithelial lesion (from Pap smear)**	
R87610	**ASC-US: atypical squamous cells of undetermined significance (from Pap smear)**	
B779	**Ascariasis unsp**	
	w/intestinal complications B770	
	w/pneumonia B7781	
	w/other complication B7789	
R188	**Ascites abdominal / NOS / pseudochylous**	
	cardiac I509 chylous (nonfilarial) I898	
	d/t alcoholic: cirrhosis K7031 hepatits K7011	
	s. japonicum B652 malignant R180 in TB A1831	
I2510	**ASCVD: arteriosclerotic cardiovascular disease non hypertensive**	
Q211	**ASD: atrial septal defect acquired ostium secundum type II**	
I25810	**ASHD: arteriosclerotic heart disease of bypass graft NOS**	
	w/unspecified angina pectoris I25799	
I25812	**ASHD: arteriosclerotic heart disease of bypass graft transplanted heart NOS**	
	w/unspecified angina pectoris I25769	
I2510	**ASHD: arteriosclerotic heart disease of native coronary artery NOS**	
	w/unspecified angina pectoris I25119	
J4520	**Asthma intermittent mild NOS**	
	w/acute exacerbation J4521	
	w/status asthmaticus J4522	
J4530	**Asthma persistent mild NOS**	
	w/acute exacerbation J4531	
	w/status asthmaticus J4532	

J4540	**Asthma persistent moderate NOS**
	w/acute exacerbation J4541
	w/status asthmaticus J4542
J4550	**Asthma persistent severe NOS**
	w/acute exacerbation J4551
	w/status asthmaticus J4552
-	**Asthma unspecified & other**
	unsp w/acute exacerbation J45901
	unsp w/status asthmaticus J45902
	unsp w/o complication J45909
	exercise induced bronchospasm J45990
	cough variant J45991
	other J45998
R279	**Ataxia NOS**
	cerebellar in other disease G3281
	cerebellar NOS / Friedreich's / early onset G111
	cerebral G3189 d/t CVA I69993
	alcoholic G312 congenital nonprogressive G110
	Ataxia-telangiectasia G118
	Marie's/primary NOS/Sanger-Brown / late onset G112
	w/defective DNA repair G113
	locomotor progressive (neurosyphilis) A5211
N170	**ATN: acute tubular necrosis NOS**
I4891	**Atrial fibrillation NOS**
	paroxysmal I480 persistent I481
	chronic I482
I4892	**Atrial flutter NOS**
	typical type I I483
	atypical type II I484
I4430	**Atrioventricular block NOS**
	1st degree I440 2nd degree I441
	complete / 3rd degree I442
	other I4439
I4430	**AVB: atrioventricular block NOS**
	complete I442
-	**Avitaminosis SEE Deficiency vitamin**
I471	**AVNRT: atrioventricular re-entrant nodal tachycardia (also AVRT)**
I471	**AVT: atrioventricular tachycardia paroxysmal (also PAT)**
R404	**Awareness altered transient**
L02411	**Axilla abscess cutaneous right, code organism if known**
	left L02412
L02431	**Axilla carbuncle right, code organism if known**
	left L02432
L02421	**Axilla furuncle/boil right**
	left L02422
L02212	**Back abscess cutaneous, code organism if known**
	any part except buttock
L02232	**Back carbuncle, code organism if known**
	any part except buttock

L02222	**Back furuncle/boil, code organism if known**	
	any part except buttock	
L89149	**Back pressure ulcer left lower NOS**	
	unstageable L89140	
	stage 1 L89141 stage 2 L89142	
	stage 3 L89143 stage 4 L89144	
L89129	**Back pressure ulcer left upper NOS**	
	unstageable L89120	
	stage 1 L89121 stage 2 L89122	
	stage 3 L89123 stage 4 L89124	
L89139	**Back pressure ulcer right lower NOS**	
	unstageable L89130	
	stage 1 L89131 stage 2 L89132	
	stage 3 L89133 stage 4 L89134	
L89119	**Back pressure ulcer right upper NOS**	
	unstageable L89110	
	stage 1 L89111 stage 2 L89112	
	stage 3 L89113 stage 4 L89114	
L89109	**Back pressure ulcer unspecified area NOS**	
	unstageable L89100	
	stage 1 L89101 stage 2 L89102	
	stage 3 L89103 stage 4 L89104	
-	**Back ulcer non-pressure chronic NOS**	
	limited to skin: L98421	
	fat layer exposed: L98422	
	muscle necrosis: L98423	
	bone necrosis: L98424	
	NOS: unsp L98429	
M549	**Backache NOS**	
R7881	**Bacteremia NOS code organism if known**	
N390	**Bacteriuria NOS**	
J45901	**BAIAE: bronchial asthma in acute exacerbation**	
M7120	**Baker's cyst (knee) unsp**	
	right M7121 left M7122	
N481	**Balanitis NOS**	
	xerotica obliterans N480	
	candidal balanitis B3742	
	gonococcal balanitis A5423	
	herpesviral [herpes simplex] balanitis A6001	
N750	**Bartholin's gland cyst (also duct cyst)**	
F458	**BBS: bashful bladder syndrome**	
M352	**Behcet's syndrome**	
	RELATED Vulva ulceration N770	
G510	**Bell's palsy**	
E5111	**Beriberi NOS**	
	wet/ cardiovascular E5112	
	RELATED Polyneuropathy G63	
K4020	**BIH: bilateral inguinal hernia NOS -- SEE INGUINAL HERNIA FOR MORE**	
	recurrent K4021	

K838	**Bile duct adhesions/atrophy/hypertrophy/ulcer**
K8050	**Bile duct calculus / choledolithiasis NOS**
	obstructed K8051
K8030	**Bile duct calculus w/cholangitis NOS**
	w/cholangitis obstructed K8031
	w/acute cholangitis NOS K8032 obstructed K8033
	w/chronic cholangitis NOS K8034 obstructed K8035
	w/acute & chronic cholangits NOS K8036 obstructed K8037
K839	**Bile duct disease NOS**
	adhesions/atrophy/hypertrophy/ulcer K838
	obstruction K831 perforation K832
	fistula K833 cyst K835
	cholangitis NOS K830
K745	**Biliary cirrhosis NOS**
	primary K743
	secondary K744
K835	**Biliary tract cyst**
J672	**Bird fancier's lung**
R55	**Blackout NOS**
N3080	**Bladder abscess NOS**
	w/hematuria N3081
N312	**Bladder atony**
N3289	**Bladder calcified / contracted**
N210	**Bladder calculus**
-	**Bladder catheter complication**
	mechanical breakdown: cystostomy T83010- other T83018-
	displacement: cystostomy T83020- other T83028-
	leakage: cystostomy T83030- other T83038-
	other mechanical: cystostomy T83090- other T83098-
	infection/ inflammation T8351X-
	7th character indicates encounter
	A - initial encounter D - subsequent encounter S - sequela
Z466	**Bladder catheter fitting & adjustment**
G9589	**Bladder cord NOS**
N329	**Bladder disorder NOS**
N3289	**Bladder disorder other**
	includes hemorrhage, hypertrophy, calcified, contracted
N323	**Bladder diverticulum**
N319	**Bladder dysfunction neurogenic / neuromuscular NOS**
R3914	**Bladder emptying incomplete**
	if applicable/known code cause first
N808	**Bladder endometriosis**
N3010	**Bladder fibrosis interstitial**
R934	**Bladder filling defect (found on imaging)**
N322	**Bladder fistula NOS**
D494	**Bladder growth NOS**
N3289	**Bladder hemorrhage NOS**
N312	**Bladder high compliance**
N3281	**Bladder hyperactivity/hypertonicity / overactive**

N3289	**Bladder hyperemia**
R32	**Bladder incontinence NOS**

    functional R3981 post-void dribbling N3943
    stress N393 urge N3941
    w/o sensory awareness N3942
    nocturnal enuresis N3944
    continuous leakage N3945 mixed N3946
    overflow N39490
    other / total / reflex N39498

-	**BLADDER INFECTION -- SEE CYSTITIS**
N319	**Bladder instability**
N318	**Bladder low compliance**
N320	**Bladder neck contracture / obstruction / stenosis acquired**
-	**Bladder neoplasm Malignant primary**

    trigone C670   dome C671
    lateral wall C672   anterior wall C673
    posterior wall C674   neck C675
    ureteric orifice C676 urachus C677
    overlapping sites C678   unsp / NOS C679
    Secondary C7911   Benign D303
    Mets to bone C7951   mets to unsp lymph nodes C779

N319	**Bladder neurogenic NOS**

    d/t cauda equina syndrome G834
    cord bladder NOS G9589

-	**Bladder neuropathic NEC**

    uninhibited N310
    reflex N311
    flaccid N312

N3281	**Bladder overactive**
N8110	**Bladder prolapse female NOS**

    midline N8111   lateral N8112

H01009	**Blepharitis NOS**

    upper lid: right H01001 left H01004
    lower lid: right H01002 left H01005
    unsp lid: right HO1003 left H01006
    Change 5th character if type known:
    Ulcerative blepharitis = 1
    Squamous blepharitis = 2

G245	**Blepharospasm NOS**

    d/t drugs G2401

K902	**Blind Loop syndrome NOS**

    postop K912

-	**Blindness**
	both eyes H540
	blind one eye low vision other unsp H5410
	blind right eye low vision left eye H5411
	blind left eye low vision right eye H5412
	blind one eye unspec H5450
	blind right eye normal vision left H5441
	blind left eye normal vision right H5442
	legal blindness H548
R140	**Bloating**
-	**Blood Cell Count - SEE RBC or WBC**
K921	**Blood in stool (melena)**
	occult blood R195
-	**Blood pressure elevated diagnosis - SEE Hypertension**
R030	**Blood pressure elevated w/o diagnosis of hypertension**
R031	**Blood pressure reading low NOS**
R6889	**Blood pressure unstable**
-	**Blood sugar SEE Glucose**
D892	**BMH: benign monoclonal hypergammaglobulinemia**
	polyclonal (Waldenström) D890
R948	**BMR: basal metabolic rate abnormal**
N320	**BNO: bladder neck obstruction (acquired)**
	congenital Q6431
-	**Boil - SEE furuncle at site**
M8560	**Bone cyst degenerative/NOS unsp site**
	aneurysmal/solitary/unicameral unsp site M8540
M8700	**Bone necrosis aseptic/avascular NOS unsp bone**
	SEE osteonecrosis at arm or leg
C7951	**Bone neoplasm SECONDARY / Mets to bone**
	to bone marrow C7952
M779	**Bone spur NOS**
	Calcaneal spur unsp foot M7730
	Calcaneal spur right foot M7731
	Calcaneal spur left foot M7732
	Iliac crest spur unsp hip M7620
	Iliac crest spur right hip M7621
	Iliac crest spur left hip M7622
	vertebrae spur M2578
J8489	**BOOP: bronchiolitis obliterans organizing pneumonia**
K550	**Bowel ischemia / infarction / necrosis acute**
-	**BOWEL -- ALSO see colon**
R194	**Bowel habit change NOS**
K5641	**Bowel impaction fecal**
	other K5649
K589	**Bowel irritable NOS (IBS)**
	w/diarrhea K580
K592	**Bowel neurogenic NOS**

K5660	**Bowel obstruction NOS**

        other / obstructive ileus/ stenosis NOS   K5669
        postoperative K913

K560	**Bowel paralytic ileus**
-	**Bowel sounds**

        absent R1911
        hyperactive R1912
        abnormal NOS R1915

K562	**Bowel volvulus**

        incl strangulation, torsion, twist

N400	**BPH: benign prostatic hypertrophy NOS**

        with lower urinary tract symptoms (LUTS) N401 Also code LUTS

H8110	**BPPV: benign positional paroxysmal vertigo NOS unsp**

        bilat H8113   right ear H8111 left ear H8112

Z4689	**Brace orthopedic fitting & adjustment**
R001	**Bradycardia NOS**
G060	**Brain abscess and/or granuloma NOS**

        in TB A1781   amebic A066
        chromomycotic B431
        gonococcal A5482

N61	**Breast abscess acute/chronic/nonpuerperal**
N6089	**Breast cyst sebaceous NOS**

        solitary N6009
        cystic/fibrocystic N6019
        Change final character if breast is known
        right =1 left = 2

N6029	**Breast fibroadenosis unsp**

        right N6021   left N6022

N6019	**Breast fibrocystic unsp**

        right N6011   left N6012

N6039	**Breast fibrosclerosis unsp**

        right N6031   left N6032

N63	**Breast lesion/lump/mass NOS**
-	**Breast neoplasm female (code for male = change 5th character to 2)**

        MALIGNANT Primary
        nipple & areola: unsp C50019 right C50011 left C50012
        central portion: unsp C50119 right C50111 left C50112
        upper inner quad: unsp C50219 right C50211   left C50212
        lower inner quad: unsp C50319 right C50311 left C50312
        upper outer quad: unsp C50419 right C50411 left C50412
        lower outer quad: unsp C50519 right C50511 left C50512
        axillary tail: unsp C50619 right C50611   left C50612
        overlapping sites: unsp C50819 right C50811 left C50812
        unsp site: unsp C50919 right C50911 left C50912

-	**Breast neoplasm Secondary and benign (female or male)**

        Secondary any site C7981
        benign: unsp D249 right D241   left D242
        Mets to axilla / arm lymph node   C773

N644	**Breast pain NOS**

Z4430	**Breast prosthesis fitting & adjustment NOS**

    right Z4431   left Z4432

- **Broad ligament disorders**
  - cyst N838
  - disorder noninflammatory N839
  - endometriosis N803
  - hematoma N837
  - laceration syndrome N838

- **Broad ligament neoplasm**
  - MALIGNANT primary
  - unsp C5710   right C5711   left C5712
  - Secondary C7982
  - Benign D282
  - Mets to bone C7951   mets to unsp lymph nodes C779
  - Mets to intraabdominal lymph node C772
  - Mets to intrapelvic lymph node C775

J479 **Bronchiectasis NOS**
    w/acute lower resp infection J470
    w/acute exacerbation J471

J219 **Bronchiolitis ACUTE unsp**
    d/t respiratory synctial virus J210
    d/t human metapneumovirus J211
    d/t other specified organism J218

J209 **Bronchitis acute NOS**
    Mycoplasma pneumoniae J200 Hemophilus influenzae J201
    streptococcus J202 coxsackie virus J203
    parainfluenza virus J204 respiratory syncytial virus J205
    rhinovirus J206 echovirus J207
    other specified organisms J208

J42 **Bronchitis chronic NOS**
    chronic simple J410
    chronic mucopurulent J411
    chronic mixed simple mucopurulent J418

J40 **Bronchitis NOS**

- **Bronchitis RELATED codes**
  - RELATED hx of tobacco use Z87.891 tobacco use Z72.0
  - RELATED exp to environmental smoke NOS Z77.22
  - RELATED exp to environmental smoke occupational Z57.31

J984 **Broncholithiasis**

J9801 **Bronchospasm acute**
    exercise induced J45990
    w/bronchitis code bronchitis
    w/acute bronchiolitis code bronchiolitis

G8381 **Brown-Sequard syndrome**

A239	**Brucellosis NOS**
	d/t Brucella melitensis A230
	d/t Brucella abortus A231
	d/t Brucella suis A232
	d/t Brucella canis A233
	Other A238
I820	**Budd-Chiari syndrome**
F502	**Bulemia nervosa / NOS**
I454	**Bundle branch block NOS -- SEE heart block for more**
I453	**Bundle branch block trifascicular -- SEE heart block for more**
M719	**Bursitis NOS**
L0231	**Buttock abscess cutaneous**
L0233	**Buttock carbuncle**
L0232	**Buttock furuncle/boil**
L89329	**Buttock pressure ulcer left NOS**
	unstageable L89320
	stage 1 L89321 stage 2 L89322
	stage 3 L89323 stage 4 L89324
L89319	**Buttock pressure ulcer right NOS**
	unstageable L89310
	stage 1 L89311 stage 2 L89312
	stage 3 L89313 stage 4 L89314
L89309	**Buttock pressure ulcer unspecified side NOS**
	unstageable L89300
	stage 1 L89301 stage 2 L89302
	stage 3 L89303 stage 4 L89304
L98419	**Buttock ulcer non-pressure chronic NOS**
	limited to skin L98411
	w/fat layer exposed L98412
	w/muscle necrosis L98413
	w/bone necrosis L98414
Z951	**CABG status**
R64	**Cachexia NOS Code underlying condition first if known**
	of old age R54
I2510	**CAD: coronary artery disease NOS**
E8350	**Calcium metabolism disorder NOS**
	hypocalcemia E8351
	hypercalcemia E8352
	other E8359
L97229	**Calf ulcer non-pressure chronic left NOS**
	limited to skin L97221
	w/fat layer exposed L97222
	w/muscle necrosis L97223
	w/bone necrosis L97224
L97219	**Calf ulcer non-pressure chronic right NOS**
	limited to skin L97211
	w/fat layer exposed L97212
	w/muscle necrosis L97213
	w/bone necrosis L97214

L97209	**Calf ulcer non-pressure chronic unspecified side NOS**
	limited to skin L97201
	w/fat layer exposed L97202
	w/muscle necrosis L97203
	w/bone necrosis L97204
B379	**Candidiasis NOS**
	esophagus B3781 lung B371
	vagina/vulva B373
	disseminated/systemic/sepsis B377
	skin/nails B372 stomatitis/oral B370
	ear/ otitis B3784 proctitis B3782
	meningitis B375 endocarditis B376
	cheilitis B3783 other / osteomyelitis B3789
K120	**Canker sore**
H9325	**CAPD: central auditory processing disorder**
M779	**Capsulitis NOS**
I499	**Cardiac arrythmia / dysrhythmia NOS**
T827XX-	**Cardiac device internal infected NOS**
	infected cardiac valve prosthesis T826xx-
	7th character indicates encounter
	A - initial encounter D - subsequent encounter S - sequela
I517	**Cardiac dilatation / hypertrophy NOS**
I509	**Cardiac failure NOS**
R012	**Cardiac friction fremitus / precordial friction**
	also dullness
I97111	**Cardiac insufficiency postop NOS**
	following cardiac surgery I97110
I249	**Cardiac ischemia acute NOS**
R011	**Cardiac murmur**
Z950	**Cardiac pacemaker dependence**
I510	**Cardiac septal defect acquired as sequelae to myocardial infarction old**
I517	**Cardiomegaly**
I429	**Cardiomyopathy NOS**
	Congestive I420 ischemic I255
	obstructive hypertrophic I421 other hyertrophic I422
	endomyocardial/eosinophilic I423
	congenital I424 alcoholic I426
	constrictive NOS I425 other I428
	d/t drug/external agent I427
	stress induced I5181
I5189	**Carditis NOS**
	rheumatic: acute I019 NOS I099
	coxsackie virus NOS B3320
	meningococcal NOS A3950
Z515	**Care palliative**
Z742	**Caregiver not available**
I720	**Carotid artery aneurysm**
I7771	**Carotid artery dissection**
G451	**Carotid artery insufficiency**

I6529	**Carotid artery occlusion / stenosis NOS**
	right I6521 left I6522
	bilat I6423
G9001	**Carotid sinus syncope / syndrome**
G5600	**Carpal tunnel syndrome NOS**
	right arm G5601 left arm G5602
-	**Cast ulcer SEE pressure ulcer at site**
-	**Cataract age related**
	morgagnian unsp H2520 bilat H2523
	morgagnian right H2521 left H2522
	nuclear unsp H2510 bilat H2513
	nuclear right H2511 left H2512
	combined types unsp H25819 bilat H25813
	combined typed right H25811 left H25812
	cortical unsp H25019 bilat H25013
	cortical right H25011 left H25012
	anterior subcapsular unsp H25039 bilat H25033
	anterior subcapsular right H25031 left H25032
H269	**Cataract NOS**
	drug induced unsp H2630 bilat H2633
	drug induced right H2631 left H2632
	unspecified traumatic unsp H26109 bilat H26103
	unspecified traumatic right H26101 left H26102
-	**Catheter central venous, infection d/t**
	systemic infection T80211-
	local infection T80212-
	other spec T80218-
	unsp T80219-
	7th character indicates encounter
	A - initial encounter D - subsequent encounter S - sequela
	includes Hickman, PIC, portacath, triple lumen etc
-	**Catheter fitting & adjustment**
	vascular Z452
	nonvascular Z4682
	extracorporeal dialysis Z4901
	peritoneal dialysis Z4902
G834	**Cauda equina syndrome**
-	**Causalgia SEE arm or leg**
F09	**CBS: chronic brain syndrome**
N3020	**CC: chronic cystitis NOS**
	w/hematuria N3021
	chronic interstitial NOS N3010
	chronic interstitial w/hematuria N3011
I774	**Celiac artery compression syndrome**
K900	**Celiac disease**
I671	**Cerebral aneurysm NOS nonruptured**
I670	**Cerebral artery dissection nonruptured**
I6619	**Cerebral artery occlusion & stenosis w/o infarction Anterior NOS**
	right I6611 left I6612 bilat I6613

I6609	**Cerebral artery occlusion & stenosis w/o infarction Middle NOS**
	right I6601 left I6602 bilat I6603
I669	**Cerebral artery occlusion & stenosis w/o infarction NOS**
	other I668
I6629	**Cerebral artery occlusion & stenosis w/o infarction Posterior NOS**
	right I6621 left I6622 bilat I6623
-	**Cerebral artery syndrome**
	middle G460
	anterior G461
	posterior G462
I672	**Cerebral atherosclerosis**
G936	**Cerebral edema**
I619	**Cerebral hemorrhage unsp**
I6340	**Cerebral infarction d/t cerebral artery EMBOLISM NOS**
	middle: right I63411 left I63412 NOS I63419
	anterior: right I63421 left I63422 NOS I63429
	posterior: right I63431 left I63432 NOS I63439
	cerebellar: right I63441 left I63442 NOS I63449
I6350	**Cerebral infarction d/t cerebral artery OCCLUSION / STENOSIS NOS**
	middle: right I63511 left I63512 NOS I63519
	anterior: right I63521 left I63522 NOS I63529
	posterior: right I63531 left I63532 NOS I63539
	cerebellar: right I63541 left I63542 NOS I63549
I6330	**Cerebral infarction d/t cerebral artery THROMBOSIS NOS**
	middle: right I63311 left I63312 NOS I63319
	anterior: right I63321 left I63322 NOS I63329
	posterior: right I63331 left I63332 NOS I63339
	cerebellar: right I63341 left I63342 NOS I63349
I6310	**Cerebral infarction d/t precerebral artery EMBOLISM NOS**
	vertebral artery: right I63111 left I63112 NOS I63119
	carotid artery: right I63131 left I63132 NOS I63139
	basilar artery I6312 other I6319
I6320	**Cerebral infarction d/t precerebral artery OCCLUSION / STENOSIS NOS**
	vertebral artery: right I63211 left I63.212 NOS I63219
	carotid artery: right I63231 left I63232 NOS I63239
	basilar artery I6322 other I6329
I6300	**Cerebral infarction d/t precerebral artery THROMBOSIS NOS**
	vertebral artery: right I63011 left I63012 NOS I63019
	carotid artery: right I63031 left I63032 NOS I63039
	basilar artery I6302 other I6309
I69359	**Cerebral infarction late effect hemiplegia NOS**
	dominant side: right I69351 left I69352
	nondominant side right I59353 left I69354
I639	**Cerebral infarction NOS**
	other NEC I638
	d/t cerebral venous thrombosis nonpyogenic I636
	d/t occlusion NOS I6359

I6930	**Cerebral infarction sequelae NOS (sequelae to stroke NOS)**
	aphasia I69320 dysphasia I69321
	dysarthria I69322 fluency disorder I69323
	apraxia I69390 dysphagia I69391
	facial weakness/droop I69392 ataxia I69393
	cognitive deficits I6931
I6782	**Cerebral ischemia**
G809	**Cerebral palsy NOS**
	spastic quadriplegic G800
	spastic diplegic G801
	spastic hemiplegic G802
	athetoid G803 ataxic G804 other G808
I6990	**Cerebrovascular disease late effect NOS**
	aphasia I69920 apraxia I69990
	ataxia I69993 cognitive I6991
	dysphagia I69991 dysphasia I69923 fluency
	facial weakness I69992
	vertigo, sensation, vision I69998
I6781	**Cerebrovascular insufficiency acute**
H6120	**Cerumen impacted unsp**
	right H6121 left H6122 bilat H6123
M5382	**Cervical syndrome acute (spine)**
M542	**Cervicalgia NOS**
N72	**Cervicitis**
A5403	**Cervicitis gonococcal**
Z90710	**Cervix absence w/ absence of uterus acquired**
	w/ remaining uterus Z90712
N881	**Cervix adhesions/bands**
	incl cicatrix (old postpartum)
N888	**Cervix disorder noninflammatory other**
	also atrophy / cyst / fibrosis
	unspecified noninflammatory cervix disorder N889
N879	**Cervix dysplasia NOS**
	mild (CIN type I) N870
	moderate (CIN type II) N871
	CIN type III D069
N86	**Cervix ectropion/erosion/eversion**
	aka trophic ulcer
N884	**Cervix elongation hypertrophic**
N800	**Cervix endometriosis**
N888	**Cervix fibrosis**
N883	**Cervix incompetence**

-	**Cervix neoplasm**
	MALIGNANT primary
	endocervix C530 exocervix C531
	overlapping sites C538
	unsp / NOS C539
	Secondary C7982
	Benign C260
	Mets to bone C7951 mets to unsp lymph nodes C779
	Mets to intraabdominal lymph node C772
	Mets to intrapelvic lymph node C775
N841	**Cervix polyp mucous / NOS**
N882	**Cervix stenosis/stricture**
N812	**Cervix stump prolapse**
E849	**CF: cystic fibrosis NOS**
	pulmonary E840
	intestinal except meconium E8419
	meconium ileus E8411 other E848
R5382	**CFS: chronic fatigue syndrome**
	postviral fatigue syndrome G933
G44009	**CHA: cluster headache NOS (also just CH)**
B571	**Chagas' disease acute NOS**
	acute w/heart involvement B570
	chronic w/heart involvement B572
	w/digestive system involvement unsp B5730
	w/megaesophagus B5731 w/megacolon B5732
	w/other digestive system involvement B5739
	w/nervous system involvement, unspec B5740
	w/meningitis B5741 w/meningoencephalitis B5742
	w/other nervous system involvement B5749
	w/ organ involvement other B575
Q249	**CHD: congenital heart disease NOS**
Z5111	**Chemotherapy antineoplastic as reason for visit**
T814XX-	**Chest tube site infection NOS**
	7th character indicates encounter
	A - initial encounter D - subsequent encounter S - sequela
I509	**CHF: congestive heart failure NOS**
	SEE Heart failure congestive for more
A980	**CHF: Congo/Crimean hemorrhagic fever (Congo virus)**
S069X9-	**CHI: closed head injury unspecified nature NOS**
	no LOC S069X0-
	LOC =< 30 min S069X1-
	LOC 31-59 min S069X2-
	LOC 1-5 hrs S069X3-
	7th character indicates encounter
	A - initial encounter D - subsequent encounter S - sequela

B019	**Chickenpox NOS**
	w/complication other B0189
	w/encephalitis B0111 w/meningitis B010
	w/pneumonia B012 w/myelitis B0112
	w/keratitis B0181
R6883	**Chills NOS**
	w/fever R509
K830	**Cholangitis acute/ chronic/ primary/ NOS/ recurrent/suppurative**
	chronic nonsuppurative destructive K743
K819	**Cholecystitis NOS**
	acute K810 chronic K811
	acute with chronic K812
K8020	**Cholelithiasis NOS**
	obstructed K8021
K8000	**Cholelithiasis w/acute cholecystitis NOS**
	obstructed K8001
	w/chronic cholecystis: NOS K8010 obstructed K8011
	w/chronic & acute cholecystitis: NOS K8012 obstructed K8013
	w/other cholecystitis: NOS K8018 obstructed K8019
H61039	**Chondritis ear external NOS**
	right H61031 left H61032
	bilat H61033
G255	**Chorea other / NOS**
	drug induced G254
R5382	**Chronic fatigue syndrome chronic NOS**
I898	**Chylous ascites / cyst**
G6181	**CIDP: chronic inflammatory demyelinating polyneuropathy**
N879	**CIN: cervix interstitial neoplasia NOS histologically confirmed**
	type I mild N870
	type II moderate N871
	type III D069
K0530	**CIPD: chronic inflammatory periodontal disease NOS**
	localized K0531 generalized K0532
A8100	**CJD: Creutzfeldt-Jakob disease NOS**
	familial, iatrogenic specified NEC A8109
	variant A8101
A8101	**CJDv: Creutzfeldt-Jakob disease variant (v may also be at beginning)**
N189	**CKD: chronic kidney disease NOS**
	stage I N181 stage II (mild) N182
	stage III (moderate) N183 stage IV (severe) N184
	stage V N185
	stage V requiring chronic dialysis (ESRD) N186
I739	**Claudication intermittent NOS**
	w/atherosclerosis of the extremities NOS I70219
	w/atherosclerosis of leg: right I70211 left I70212 bilat I70213
R294	**Clicking hip**
C9110	**CLL: chronic lymphoid leukemia NOS**
	in remission C9111 in relapse C9112
G600	**CMT: Charcot-Marie-Tooth disease**

B259	**CMV: cytomegalic virus local/systemic infection NOS**
	pneumonitis B250 hepatitis B251
	pancreatitis B252 other B258
	mononucleosis NOS B2710
	mono w/polyneuropathy B2711
	mono w/meningitis B271
	mono w/ other complication NEC B2719
J678	**Coffee worker's lung**
R41844	**Cognitive deficit -- executive function**
	attention / concentration deficit R41840
	communicative deficit R41841
	visuospatial deficit R41842
	psychomotor deficit R41843
	borderline intellectual function R4183
R4182	**Cognitive function altered NOS**
	age-related decline R4181
G3184	**Cognitive impairment mild, so stated**
J00	**Cold common**
J449	**COLD: chronic obstructive lung/pulmonary disease NOS (COPD)**
	includes w/asthma, bronchitis NOS, and emphysema
	w/acute lower resp infection J440
	w/acute exacerbation J441
R1084	**Colic NOS adult**
A09	**Colitis infectious/septic/ presumed infectious NOS**
	amebic nondysenteric A062
	C. dificile A047
	protozoal NOS A079
	pseudomembranous A047
K559	**Colitis ischemic NOS**
	acute K550
	chronic K551
K5150	**Colitis left sided NOS**
	w/rectal bleeding K51511
	w/intestinal obstruction K51512
	w/fistula K51513
	w/abscess K51514
	other spec complicaton K51518
	w/unsp complication K51519
K529	**Colitis noninfective NOS**
	granulomatous/regional/transmural K5010 (Crohn's)
	d/t radiation K520
	eosinophilic K5282
	adaptive/membranous/mucous K589
	allergic / dietetic K522 drug induced / toxic K521

K5190	**Colitis ulcerative NOS**
	w/rectal bleeding K51911
	w/intestinal obstruction K51912
	w/fistula K51913
	w/abscess K51914
	w/other spec complication K51918
	w/unsp complication K51919
	RELATED arthritis or polyarthritis M0200
M359	**Collagen disease NOS/non vascular**
	vascular M310
-	**Colles' fracture (radius)**
	unsp S52539- right S52531- left S52532-
	7th character indicates encounter/status
	A - initial
	D - subsequent routine healing
	G - subsequent delayed healing
	K - subsequent nonunion
	P - subsequent malunion
	S - sequela
K630	**Colon abscess**
K660	**Colon adhesions**
K598	**Colon atonic/atony**
K593	**Colon dilatation**
-	**Colon diverticular disease**
	diverticulitis w/perforation & abscess K5720
	diverticulitis w/perforation & abscess w/bleeding K5721
	diverticulitis: NOS K5732 w/bleeding K5733
	diverticulosis NOS K5730
	diverticulosis w/bleeding K5731
N805	**Colon endometriosis**
K5010	**Colon enteritis regional NOS**
	SEE Crohn's disease large intestine for more
K632	**Colon fistula NOS**
K560	**Colon ileus paralytic**
K5641	**Colon impaction fecal**
	other K5649
K561	**Colon intussusception/invagination**
K589	**Colon irritable**
	w/diarrhea K580
K550	**Colon ischemia / infarction / necrosis acute**

-	**Colon neoplasm**
	MALIGNANT primary
	cecum C180 appendix C181
	ascending colon C182 hepatic flexure C183
	transverse colon C184 splenic flexure C185
	descending colon C186 sigmoid colon C187
	overlapping sites C188 unspecified C189
	SECONDARY C785
	BENIGN cecum D120 appendix D121 ascending colon D122
	transverse colon D123 descending colon D124
	sigmoid colon D125 unsp/NOS D126
K592	**Colon neurogenic**
K5669	**Colon obstruction/occlusion/stenosis/stricture other**
	unsp obstruction K5660
-	**Colon paralysis**
	K560
K631	**Colon perforation nontraumatic**
Z86010	**Colon polyp history**
K635	**Colon polyp NOS**
	Adenomatous polyp / polyposis D126
	Inflammatory NOS K5140
	Inflammatory w/ rectal bleeding K51411
	Inflammatory w/ intestinal obstruction K51412
	Inflammatory w/ fistula K51413
	Inflammatory w/ abscess K51414
	Inflammatory w/ other complication K51418
	Inflammatory w/ unspecified complications K51419
K589	**Colon spastic**
	w/diarrhea K580
K562	**Colon volvulus**
	incl strangulation, torsion, twist
Z433	**Colostomy care, closure/takedown, toilet/cleansing**
	status w/o need for care Z933
	fitting & adjust Z4659
K9400	**Colostomy complication NOS**
	hemorrhage K9401 malfunction K9403
	other K9409 infection K9402
	for infection also code type eg. abd wall cellulitis L03311 or a sepsis
	granulation of surrounding skin L928
-	**Compartment syndrome nontraumatic**
	unsp or other M79A9 abdomen M79A3
	Leg: unsp M79A29 right M79A21 left M79A22
	Arm: unsp M79A19 right M79A11 left M79A12
R410	**Confusion**
F05	**Confusion organic acute/subacute/NOS**
I509	**Congestive heart failure NOS**
	SEE heart failure congestive for more

B309	**Conjunctivitis viral NOS**
	keratoconjunctivitis d/t adenovirus B300
	conjunctivitis d/t adenovirus B301
	pharyngoconjunctivitis B302
	acute epidemic hemorrhagic conjunctivitis B303
	other / Newcastle B308
K5900	**Constipation NOS**
	slow transit K5901
	outlet dysfunction K5902
	other K5909
	fecal impaction K5641
	incomplete defecation R150
	psychogenic F458
M2450	**Contractures NOS**
	SEE site if known
Z5189	**Convalescence following radiotherapy**
R569	**Convulsions NOS**
	febrile NOS R5600 febrile complex R5601
	post traumatic R561
R279	**Coordination lack of NOS**
	ataxia NOS R270
	other R278
I2609	**Cor pulmonale acute NOS**
	chronic/NOS I2781
	acute w/saddle embolus of pulmonary artery I2602
	acute w/septic pulmonary embolism I2601
G9589	**Cord bladder NOS**
E7403	**Cori disease**
I2510	**Coronary artery atherosclerosis native artery NOS**
	w/unstable angina I25110
	w/angina & documented spasm I25111
	w/other angina I25118
	w/unspecified angina I25119
	RELATED
	atherosclerosis d/t lipid rich plaque I2583
	atherosclerosis d/t calcified coronary lesion I2584
Z951	**Coronary artery bypass graft status**
I2542	**Coronary artery dissection**
-	**Coronary artery occlusion**
	chronic total occlusion I2582
	acute not resulting in MI I240
R05	**Cough NOS**
	psychogenic F458
	smoker's J410
	w/hemorrhage NOS R042
N340	**Cowper's gland abscess**
B3322	**Coxsackie virus myocarditis**

G809	**CP: cerebral palsy NOS**
	mixed / other G808
	spastic quadriplegic G800
	spastic diplegic (spastic NOS) G801
	spastic hemiplegic G802
	athetoid G803 ataxic G804
G890	**CPS: central pain syndrome**
R252	**Cramp in limbs NOS**
	charley-horse M62831
	muscle spasm of back M62830
	carpopedal spasm R290
	cramps leg sleep related G4762
T672XXA	**Cramps heat**
	7th character indicates encounter
	A - initial encounter D - subsequent encounter S - sequela
T80211	**CRBSI: catheter related blood stream infection - also code specified infection**
N189	**CRD: chronic renal disease NOS**
	stage 1 N181 stage 2 N182
	stage 3 N183 stage 4 N184
	stage 5 N185 end stage N186
A8100	**Creutzfeldt-Jakob disease NOS**
	other A8109
	variant A8101
	RELATED dementia F2080 w/ behavioral disturbance F0281
N189	**CRF: chronic renal failure NOS - SEE CRD for more**
N189	**CRI: chronic renal insufficiency - SEE CRD for more**
K50819	**Crohn's disease both large & small intestine complicated NOS**
	w/rectal bleeding K50811
	w/intestinal obstruction K50812
	w/fistula K50813 w/abscess K50814
	w/other complication K50818
K5080	**Crohn's disease both large & small intestine NOS**
K50119	**Crohn's disease large intestine complicated NOS**
	w/rectal bleeding K50111
	w/intestinal obstruction K50112
	w/fistula K50113 w/abscess K50114
	w/other complication K50118
K5010	**Crohn's disease large intestine NOS**
K50019	**Crohn's disease small intestine complicated NOS**
	w/rectal bleeding K50011
	w/intestinal obstruction K50012
	w/fistula K50013 w/abscess K50014
	w/other complication K50018
K5000	**Crohn's disease small intestine NOS**

K50919	**Crohn's disease unsp intestine complicated NOS**
	w/rectal bleeding K50911
	w/intestinal obstruction K50912
	w/fistula K50913 w/abscess K50914
	w/other complication K50918
K5090	**Crohn's disease unspec intestine NOS**
R7982	**CRP: c-reactive protein elevated**
-	**CRPS: complex regional pain syndrome**
	CRPS I
	arm: right G90511 left G90512 bilat G90513 NOS G90519
	leg: right G90521 left G90522 bilat G90523 NOS G90529
	other site G9059 unsp G9050
	CRPS II
	leg: right G5771 left G5772 NOS G5770
	arm: right G5641 left G5642 NOS G5640
M341	**CRST: calcinosis Raynauds sclerodactyltelangiectasis also CREST**
G4731	**CSA: central sleep apnea primary**
	in other conditions G4737
G5600	**CTS: carpal tunnel syndrome NOS**
	right G5601 left G5602
E249	**Cushing's syndrome NOS**
	pituitary dependent E240 drug induced E242
	alcohol induced pseudo E244 other E248
	Nelson's syndrome E241
	ectopic ACTH syndrome E243
-	**CVA late effect monoplegia**
	unspec side: arm I69339 leg I69349
	dominant arm: right I69331 left I69332
	nondominant arm: right I69.333 left I69.334
	dominant leg: right I69.341 left I69.342
	nondominant leg: right I69.343 left I69.344
Z8673	**CVA: cerebrovascular accident - history**
I639	**CVA: cerebrovascular accident acute/NOS (stroke)**
R230	**Cyanosis**
E849	**Cystic fibrosis NOS**
	w/meconium ileus E8411
	other intestinal manifestations E8419
	w/other manifestations E848
	w/pulmonary manifestations E840
A5401	**Cystitis gonococcal**
-	**Cystitis w/ hematuria**
	acute N3001 interstitial chronic N3011
	other chronic N3021 trigonitis N3031
	irradiation N3041 other N3081
	NOS N3091

-	**Cystitis w/o hematuria**
	acute N3000 interstitial chronic N3010
	other chronic N3020 trigonitis N3030
	irradiation N3040 other N3080
	NOS N3090
Z435	**Cystostomy aftercare**
	aftercare for other urinary tract opening Z436
N99518	**Cystostomy complication other**
	hemorrhage N99510
	infection N99511
	malfunction N99512
Z9350	**Cystostomy status NOS**
	cutaneous-vesicostomy Z9351
	appendico-vesicostomy Z9352
	other specified Z9359
B259	**Cytomegalic virus infection NOS**
	pneumonitis B250 hepatitis B251
	pancreatitis B252 other B258
	mononucleosis NOS B2710
	mono w/polyneuropathy B2711
	mono w/meningitis B271
	mono w/ other complication NEC B2719
-	**DDD: degenerative disc disease NOS**
	lumbar M5136
	lumbosacral M5137
	thoracic M5134
	thoracolumbar M5135
R5381	**Debility NOS**
	age related R54
R29898	**Decline in function acute**
-	**DECUBITUS ULCER -- SEE pressure ulcer at site**
Z4502	**Defibrillator fitting & adjustment implantable**
E630	**Deficiency essential fatty acid**
E619	**Deficiency nutrient element NOS**
	calcium E58 selenium E59
	zinc E60 copper E610 iron E611
	magnesium E612
E639	**Deficiency nutritional NOS**
-	**Deficiency sequelae - Code first the actual sequelae**
	d/t protein-calorie malnutrition E640
	d/t vitamin A deficiency E641
	d/t vitamin C deficiency E642
	d/t rickets, vit D deficiency E643
	d/t unspecified nutrition deficiency E649
	other nutritional deficiency E648
E519	**Deficiency thiamine NOS**
	dry beriberi E5111 wet beriberi E5112
	Wernicke's encephalopathy E512
	other E518

E509	**Deficiency vitamin A NOS**
	w/conjunctival xerosis: E500 w/Bitot's spot E501
	w/corneal xerosis: E502 w/ulceration E503
	w/keratomalacia E504
	w/night blindness E505
	w/non-ocular manifestations E508
E539	**Deficiency vitamin B NOS**
	other specified B vitamins E538
	other includes biotin, folate, folic acid, pantothenic acid, B12
-	**Deficiency vitamin B12 RELATED ANEMIA**
	unsp D519
	d/t intrinsic factor deficiency D510
	d/t malabsorption D511
	transcobalamin II deficiency D512
	other dietary deficiency D513
	other deficiency D518
E530	**Deficiency vitamin B2/riboflavin**
E531	**Deficiency vitamin B6/pyridoxine**
E54	**Deficiency vitamin C**
E559	**Deficiency vitamin D NOS**
	active rickets E550
E560	**Deficiency vitamin E**
E561	**Deficiency vitamin K**
E860	**Dehydration**
F0150	**Dementia vascular unsp**
	w/behavioral disturbance F0151
Z993	**Dependence on wheelchair**
	Code cause first
F339	**Depressive disorder major recurrent episode NOS**
	mild F330 moderate F331
	severe F332 severe w/psychotic behavior F333
	in remission NOS F3340
	full remission F3342 partial remission F3341
	recurrent brief episodes F338
F329	**Depressive disorder major single episode NOS**
	mild F320 moderate F321
	severe NOS F322 severe w/psychotic behavior F323
	partial or unspecified remission F324
	in full remission F325
L239	**Dermatitis allergic CONTACT unsp**
	d/t metals L230 d/t adhesives L231
	d/t cosmetics L232 d/t drugs on skin L233
	d/t dyes L234 d/t other chemical products
	d/t food L236 d/t plants non-food L237
	d/t animal hair L2381 d/t other agent L2389
L219	**Dermatitis seborrheic NOS**
	capitis L210
	infantle L211
	other L218

L259	**Dermatitis unspecified form CONTACT unsp**
	d/t cosmetics L250 d/t drugs L251
	d/t dyes L252 d/t other chemicals L253
	d/t food on skin L254 d/t plants nonfood L255
	d/t other agents L258
-	**DHTR: delayed hemolytic transfusion reaction**
	after 24 hrs d/t Rh incompatibility T80411-
	after 24 hrs d/t ABO incompatibility T80311-
	at unspecified time d/t Rh incompatibility T80419-
	at unspecified time d/t ABO incompatibility T80319-
	7th character indicates encounter
	A - initial encounter D - subsequent encounter S - sequela
-	**Diabetes RELATED edema**
	unsp R609
	localized R600
	generalized R601
-	**Diabetes RELATED insulin and oral antidiabetic toxicity**
	accidental/NOS T383X1-
	adverse effect T383X5-
	underdosing T383X6-
	intentional self harm T383x2-
	assault T383x3-
	undetermined T383x4-
	7th character indicates encounter
	A - initial encounter D - subsequent encounter S - sequela
E1136	**Diabetes Type 2 w/complication cataract**
	drug or chemical induced E0936
-	**Diabetes Type 2 w/complication circulatory**
	peripheral angiopathy NOS E1151
	peripheral angiopathy w/gangrene E1152
	other E1159
	if specified drug or chemical induced, change '11' to '09'
E1100	**Diabetes Type 2 w/complication hyperosmolarity NOS**
	w/coma E1101
	if specified drug or chemical induced, change '11' to '09'
E11649	**Diabetes Type 2 w/complication hypoglycemia NOS**
	w/coma E11641
	if specified drug or chemical induced, change '11' to '09'
-	**Diabetes Type 2 w/complication kidney**
	w/ nephropathy / glomerulosclerosis E1121
	w/ other / tubular degeneration E1129
	w/ chronic kidney disease E1122 also code CKD
	if specified drug or chemical induced, change '11' to '09'
	Chronic kidney disease codes:
	NOS N189 stage 1 N181 stage 2 mild N182
	stage 3 moderate N183 stage 4 severe N184
	stage 5 N185 end stage N186
	For stage 6 (ESRD) also code dialysis status Z992

-	**Diabetes Type 2 w/complication neurological**
	neuropathy NOS E1140 mononeuropathy E1141
	polyneuropathy / neuralgia E1142
	autonomic polyneuropathy / gastroparesis E1143
	amyotrophy E1144 other E1149
	if specified drug or chemical induced, change '11' to '09'
-	**Diabetes Type 2 w/complication oral**
	w/periodontal disease E11630
	other oral complication E11638
	if specified drug or chemical induced, change '11' to '09'
-	**Diabetes Type 2 w/complication retinopathy nonproliferative**
	mild: NOS E11329 w/macular edema E11321
	moderate: NOS E11339 w/macular edema E11331
	severe: NOS E11349 w/macular edema E11341
	if specified drug or chemical induced, change '11' to '09'
E11319	**Diabetes Type 2 w/complication retinopathy NOS**
	w/macular edema E11311
	if specified drug or chemical induced, change '11' to '09'
E11359	**Diabetes Type 2 w/complication retinopathy proliferative NOS**
	w/macular edema E11351
	if specified drug or chemical induced, change '11' to '09'
-	**Diabetes Type 2 w/complication skin**
	dermatitis E11620 foot ulcer E11621
	other skin ulcer E11622
	other skin complication E11628
	Also code ulcers at site
	if specified drug or chemical induced, change '11' to '09'
E119	**Diabetes Type 2 w/o complication NOS**
T8571x-	**Dialysis catheter peritoneal infected**
	7th character indicates encounter
	A - initial encounter D - subsequent encounter S - sequela
R197	**Diarrhea NOS**
	chronic noninfectious K529
	functional K591 dietetic K522
	in IBS K580 drug induced K521
	amebic A060 psychogenic F458
	postpro gastrointestinal surgery k911
	other postpro K9189
	dysenteric/epidemic/infectious NOS A09
D65	**DIC: disseminated intravascular coagulopathy**
G830	**Diplegia**

M4810	**DISH: diffuse idiopathic skeletal hyperostosis NOS**
	occipito-atlanto-axial M4811
	cervical M4812
	cervicothoracic M4813
	thoracic M4814
	thoracolumbar M4815
	lumbar M4816
	lumbosacral M4817
	sacral and sacrococcygeal M4818
	multiple sites M4819
D6959	**DIT: drug induced thrombocytopenia**
R42	**Dizziness**
M1990	**DJD: degenerative joint disease NOS**
E1010	**DKA: diabetic ketoacidosis type I DM w/o coma**
	w/coma E1011
E109	**DM: diabetes mellitus type I NOS**
E119	**DM: diabetes mellitus unsp or type II NOS**
	SEE diabetes for more
A312	**DMAC: disseminated mycobacterium avium-intracellulare complex**
G241	**DMD: dystonia musculorum deformans**
-	**DME: diabetic macular edema**
	w/unspecified diabetic retinopathy E11311
	w/mild nonproliferative diabetic retinopathy E11321
	w/moderate nonproliferative diabetic retinopathy E11331
	w/severe nonproliferative diabetic retinopathy E11341
	w/proliferative diabetic retinopathy E11351
Z66	**DNR: do not resuscitate status**
-	**DRESSING CHANGE - SEE wound aftercare**
R400	**Drowsiness**
Z5181	**Drug level monitoring (therapeutic drug)**
	Also code applicable long term (current) use
-	**Drug use long term (current)**
	aspirin Z7982 other NSAID Z791
	postmenopausal hormone replacement Z79890
	insulin Z794 antibiotics Z792 anticoagulant Z7901
	opiate analgesic Z79891 antiplatelet Z7902
	hormonal contraceptives Z793
	inhaled steroids Z7951 systemic steroids Z7952
	biphosphonates Z7983
L565	**DSAP: disseminated superficial actinic porokeratosis**
-	**DSTR: delayed serologic transfusion reaction**
	d/t Rh incompatibility T8049x-
	d/t ABO incompatibility T8039x-
	unsp incompatibility T8089x-
	7th character indicates encounter
	A - initial encounter D - subsequent encounter S - sequela
F10231	**DT's: delerium tremens NOS**
K911	**Dumping syndrome**
-	**Duodenal ulcer SEE ULCER GI**

K2980	**Duodenitis NOS**
	w/bleeding K2981
K317	**Duodenum polyp**
K269	**Duodenum ulcer NOS**
	acute: w/hemorrhage K260 w/perforation K261
	acute: NOS K263 w/both hemorrhage /perforation K262
	chronic/unsp: w/hemorrhage K264 w/perforation K265
	chronic/unsp w/both hemorrhage / perforation K266
	chronic NOS K267
Z86718	**DVT personal history of deep vein thrombosis**
-	**DVT: deep vein thrombosis**
	SEE arm or leg for codes
K30	**Dyspepsia functional**
I69391	**Dysphagia following cerebral infarction**
	Also code phase of dysphagia
R1310	**Dysphagia NOS (phases)**
	oral phase R1311
	oropharyngeal phase R1312
	pharyngeal phase R1313
	pharyngoeophageal phase R1314
	other / cervical / neurogenic R1319
R4702	**Dysphasia NOS**
	d/t CVA or CVD I69921
R0600	**Dyspnea NOS**
	orthopnea R0601 shortness of breath R0602
	other forms of dyspnea R0609
G904	**Dysreflexia autonomic**
	RELATED fecal impaction K5641
	RELATED urinary tract infection N390
	RELATED pressure ulcer - SEE site
G249	**Dystonia NOS**
	idiopathic nonfamilial G242
	idiopathic orofacial G244
	other G248
	blepharospasm NOS G245
	spasmodic torticollis G243
	drug induced: subacute G2401 acute G2402 other G2409
	genetic torsion G241
R300	**Dysuria**
	painful urination NOS R309
-	**EAR INFECTION - SEE OTITIS**
-	**Ear Perichondritis SEE Perichondritis ear external**
H6120	**Ear wax impacted NOS**
	right H6121 left H6122 bilat H6123
H9209	**Earache NOS**
	right H9201 left H9202 bilat H9203

B2700	**EBV: Epstein Barr virus infection (mononucleosis) unsp**
	w/complication other B2709
	w/meningitis B2702
	w/polyneuropathy B2701
R233	**Ecchymoses spontaneous**
E8889	**ECD: Erdheim-Chester disease**
R9431	**ECG: electrocardiogram abnormal**
Z9281	**ECMO: extracorporeal membrane oxygenation personal history**
T783XX-	**Edema angioneurotic / allergic**
	7th character indicates encounter
	A - initial encounter D - subsequent encounter S - sequela
R609	**Edema NOS**
	localized NOS R600
	generalized NOS R601
	nutritional severe NOS E43
	nutritional w/dyspigmentation of skin & hair E40
	malignant A480
Q796	**EDS: Ehlers-Danlos syndrome**
R9401	**EEG: electroencephalogram abnormal NOS**
M2540	**Effusion of joint NOS**
	SEE site for more
N8502	**EIN: Endometrium intraepithelial neoplasia**
R9431	**EKG: electrocardiogram abnormal**
M24629	**Elbow ankylosis unsp**
	right M24621 left M24622
M25729	**Elbow bone spur (osteophyte) unsp**
	right M25721 left M25722
-	**Elbow bursitis**
	olecranon unsp M7020 right M7021 left M7022
	other unsp M7030 right M7031 left M7032
M71429	**Elbow calcification unsp**
	right M71421 left M71422
M94229	**Elbow chondromalacia unsp**
	right M94221 left M94222
M24529	**Elbow contractures unsp**
	right M24521 left M24522
M25429	**Elbow effusion (joint) unsp**
	right 25421 left M25422
-	**Elbow gout acute / NOS**
	idiopathic/primary right M10021 left M10022 unsp M10029
	drug induced right M10221 left M10222 unsp M10229
	d/t renal impairment right M10321 left M10322 unsp M10329
	lead induced right M10121 left M10122 unsp M10129
	other secondary right M10421 left M10422 unsp M10429

-	**Elbow gout chronic**
	idiopathic/primary right M1A021- left M1A022- unsp M1A029-
	lead induced right M1A121- left M1A122- unsp M1A129-
	drug induced right M1A221- left M1A222- unsp M1A229-
	d/t renal impairment right M1A321- left M1A322- unsp M1A329-
	other secondary right M1A421- left M1A422- unsp M1A429-
	The appropriate 7th character
	0 = without tophus (tophi) 1 = with tophus (tophi)
M25029	**Elbow hemarthrosis unsp**
	right M25021 left M25022
M24829	**Elbow joint instability NOS unsp**
	right M24821 left M24822
M24029	**Elbow joint mice unsp**
	right M24021 left M24022
M19029	**Elbow osteoarthritis primary unsp**
	right M19021 left M19022
M25529	**Elbow pain unsp**
	right M25521 left M25522
L89029	**Elbow pressure ulcer left NOS**
	unstageable L89020
	stage 1 L89021 stage 2 L89022
	stage 3 L89023 stage 4 L89024
L89019	**Elbow pressure ulcer right NOS**
	unstageable L89010
	stage 1 L89011 stage 2 L89012
	stage 3 L89013 stage 4 L89014
L89009	**Elbow pressure ulcer unsp NOS**
	unstageable L89000
	stage 1 L89001 stage 2 L89002
	stage 3 L89003 stage 4 L89004
-	**Embolism and thrombosis of deep veins SEE Arm or Leg DVT**
I423	**EMF: endomyocardial fibrosis**
J439	**Emphysema NOS**
	unilateral pulmonary J430 centrilobar J432
	panlobar J431 other J438
	RELATED hx of tobacco use Z87891 tobacco use Z720
	RELATED exp to environmental smoke NOS Z7722
	RELATED exp to environmental smoke occupational Z5731
G0400	**Encephalitis and encephalomyelitis disseminated acute NOS**
	postinfectious G0401
	postimmunization G0402
G0490	**Encephalitis and encephalomyelitis NOS**
A3981	**Encephalitis meningococcal**
B262	**Encephalitis mumps**
B050	**Encephalitis postmeasles**
B0111	**Encephalitis postvaricella / postchickenpox**
B941	**Encephalitis viral SEQUELAE**

A839	**Encephalitis viral mosquito borne NOS**
	Japanese A830
	Western equine A831
	Eastern equine A832
	St Louis A833
	Australian A834
	California A835
	Rocio viru A836
A86	**Encephalitis viral NOS**
	enteroviral A850
	adenoviral A851
	arthropod borne unsp A852
	lethargica A858
A849	**Encephalitis viral tick borne NOS**
	Far Eastern / Russian A840
	Central European A841
	other A841
A831	**Encephalitis Western equine**
I674	**Encephalopathy hypertensive**
G0430	**Encephalopathy necrotizing hemorrhagic acute NOS**
	postinfectious G0431
	postimmunization G0432
	other G0439
G3182	**Encephalopathy necrotizing subacute**
I6783	**Encephalopathy syndrome posterior reversible**
B376	**Endocarditis candidal**
I38	**Endocarditis chronic NOS**
I339	**Endocarditis subacute & acute unsp**
	infective I330
N72	**Endocervicitis**
N809	**Endometriosis unsp (see site for more)**
N719	**Endometritis unsp**
	chronic N711
	acute N710
N8500	**Endometrium hyperplasia NOS**
	benign / complex or simple w/o atypia N8501
	w/atypia N8502 (EIN)
N8502	**Endometrium intraepithelial neoplasia**
N840	**Endometrium polyp**
A049	**Enteritis bacterial NOS**
	e coli enteropathogenic A040
	e coli enterotoxigenic A041
	e coli enterohemorrhagic A043
	e coli other A044
	campylobacter A045
	c. difficile A047
	yersinia enterocolitica A046
M0210	**Enteritis infectious RELATED Arthropathy**

K559	**Enteritis ischemic NOS**
	acute K550 chronic K551
A084	**Enteritis viral NOS**
	viral Norwalk / Norwalk like agent A0811
	SRV NOS A0819 rotaviral A080
	adenoviral A082 calicivirus A0831
	coxsackie / echovirus / torovirus A0839
	astrovirus A0832
K559	**Enterocolitis NOS ischemic**
	hemorrhagic acute / necrotizing NEC K550
	pseudomembranous A047
	staphylococcal A048
	ulcerative chronic K5180
	chronic K551
R94110	**EOG: electro-oculogram function study abnormal results**
R1013	**Epigastric pain**
J0510	**Epiglottitis acute NOS**
	w/obstruction J0511
G40909	**Epilepsy unsp**
	unsp w/status epilepticus G40901
	unsp intractable G40919
	unsp intractable w/status epilepticus G40911
	grand mal NOS G40409
	grand mal w/status epilepticus G40401
	grand mal intractable G40419
	grand mal intratable w/status epilepticus G40411
R040	**Epistaxis**
R9439	**EPS: electrophysiologic studies abnormal results**
Z170	**ER+: estrogen receptor positive status**
Z171	**ER-: estrogen receptor negative status**
R94111	**ERG: electroretinogram function study abnormal results**
R142	**Eructation**
L081	**Erythrasma**
Z1612	**ESBL: Extended spectrum beta lactamase, resistance to**
K209	**Esophagitis acute/NOS**
	candidiasis B3781
	eosinophilic K200
	reflux K210
	specified not candidiasis, reflux or tuberculous K208
K9430	**Esophagostomy complication unsp**
	hemorrhage K9431 infection K9432
	malfunction K9433 other K9439
K208	**Esophagus abscess NOS**
K220	**Esophagus achalasia/ aperistalsis**
K2270	**Esophagus Barrett's**
	w/ low grade dysplasia K22710
	w/ high grade dysplasia K22711
	w/ dysplasia, unspecified K22719
B3781	**Esophagus candidiasis**

K222	**Esophagus compression/obstruction**
	incl stenosis & stricture
K224	**Esophagus dismotility**
K228	**Esophagus hemorrhage**
C159	**Esophagus neoplasm malignant primary NOS**
	MALIGNANT
	upper third C153
	middle third C154
	lower third C155
	overlapping sites C158
	Secondary C7889 Benign D130
	Mets to bone C7951 mets to unsp lymph nodes C779
	mets to inguinal nodes C774 mets to axillary nodes C773
	mets to esophageal nodes C771
K223	**Esophagus perforation/rupture**
K2210	**Esophagus ulcer**
	w/bleeding K2211
	incl Barret's ulcer / fungal / NOS /peptic
	Barret's esophagus & Barret's ulcer are different codes
I8500	**Esophagus varices NOS**
	w/bleeding I8501
	secondary: NOS I8510 w/bleeding I8511
	first code other disease if known
	RELATED many alcohol related codes, if unsp code F10988
N186	**ESRD: end stage renal disease if applicable, code first chronic hypertensive kidney disease**
L0201	**Face abscess cutaneous**
	Does not include eye area, mouth, nose
L0203	**Face carbuncle, code organism if known**
L0202	**Face furuncle / boil, code organism if known**
G519	**Facial nerve disorder NOS**
	myokymia G514
	clonic hemifacial spasm G513
	palsy G510
R29810	**Facial weakness / droop NOS**
	d/t CVA I69992
R627	**Failure to thrive (adult)**
R55	**Fainting NOS**
-	**Fall from mobility aid**
	powered wheelchair non-moving W050XX-
	motorized scooter non-moving W052XX-
	for above 7th character indicates encounter
	A - initial encounter D - subsequent encounter S - sequela
	mobility scooter moving V00831
	powered wheelchair moving V00811
Z9181	**Fall history of or at risk of**
	repeated or tendency to fall R296

W19XXX-	**Fall NOS**
	from chair W07XXX-
	from commode/toilet NOS W1811X-
	from bed W06XXX- on ramp W102XX-
	on stairs and steps W108XX-
	from sidewalk curb W101XX-
	in shower / empty bathtub W182XX-
	in filled bathtub W16212-
	7th character indicates encounter
	A - initial encounter D - subsequent encounter S - sequela
N7091	**Fallopian tube abscess unsp**
	chronic N7011
	acute/subacute N7001
N8332	**Fallopian tube atrophy**
N838	**Fallopian tube cyst**
N802	**Fallopian tube endometriosis**
N848	**Fallopian tube polyp**
N8352	**Fallopian tube torsion**
	w/torsion of ovary N8353
-	**Family history**
	sudden cardiac death Z8241
	stroke Z823
	malignant neoplasms unsp Z809
I743	**FAO: femoral artery occlusion**
R5383	**Fatigue NOS**
	chronic fatigue syndrome R5382
	post viral fatigue syndrome G933
	neoplasm related (malignant) R530 Code neoplasm first
	d/t senile debility R54
	heat fatigue T676xx-
	d/t excessive exertion T733xx-
	For codes beginning with T 7th character indicates encounter
	A - initial encounter D - subsequent encounter S - sequela
R195	**Fecal abnormalities**
	color, bulk, mucus, occult blood
K5641	**Fecal impaction**
R159	**Fecal incontinence NOS**
	incomplete R150
	smearing R151
	urgency R152
R633	**Feeding difficulties NOS**
F508	**Feeding problem psychogenic, loss of appetite**

-	**Felty's syndrome**
	NOS M0500
	shoulder: right M05011 left M05012 unsp M05019
	elbow: right M05021 left M05022 unsp M05029
	wrist: right M05031 left M05032 unsp M05039
	hand: right M05041 left M05042 unsp M05049
	hip: right M05051 left M05052 unsp M05059
	knee: right M05061 left M05062 unsp M05069
	ankle & foot: right M05071 left M05072 unsp M05079
	multiple sites M0509
-	**Femoral epiphysis slipped, upper nontraumatic**
	Acute: unsp M93003 right M93011 left M93012
	Chronic: unsp M93023 right M93021 left M93022
	Acute on chronic: unsp M93033 right M93031 left M93032
	Unsp: unsp M93003 right M93001 left 93002
R509	**Fever NOS**
	drug induced R502
	postprocedural R5082 postvaccination R5083
	w/ conditions classified elsewhere R5081
	posttransfusion R5084
A8183	**FFI: fatal familial insomnia**
M724	**Fibromatosis pseudosarcomatous**
M797	**Fibromyalgia NOS**
	also used for fibromyositis / fibrositis / myofibrositis
L03019	**Finger cellulitis unsp**
	right L03011 left L03012
-	**Finger(s) fracture pathological NOS / (in neoplastic disease below)**
	unsp M84446- right M84444- left M84445-
	7th character indicates encounter/status
	A - initial S - sequela
	D - subsequent routine healing
	G - subsequent delayed healing
	K - subsequent nonunion P - subsequent malunion
	Change 4th character to 5 for 'in neoplastic disease'
R143	**Flatulence**
-	**Flu d/t identified avian flu virus A/H5N1 (avian / bird / swine)**
	w/other respiratory manifestations J09X2
	w/gastrointestinal manifestations J09X3
	w/other manifestations J09X9
E878	**Fluid disorder/imbalance NOS**
E8770	**Fluid overload NOS**
	d/t transfusion E8771
	other E8779
R609	**Fluid retention NOS**
I773	**FMD: fibromuscular dysplasia artery**
R5084	**FNHTR: febrile nonhemolytic transfusion reaction**
L02619	**Foot abscess cutaneous unsp**
	right L02611 left L02612

	Foot ankylosis
-	right M24674 left M24675 unsp M24676
-	**Foot blister**
	right S90821- left S90822- unsp S90829-
	7th character indicates encounter
	A - initial encounter D - subsequent encounter S - sequela
L02629	**Foot boil/ furuncle unsp**
	right L02621 left L02622
M7730	**Foot bone spur calcaneal NOS**
	Calcaneal spur right foot M7731
	Calcaneal spur left foot M7732
M25776	**Foot bone spur (osteophyte) unsp**
	right M25774 left M25775
-	**Foot Charcot's joint (and ankle)**
	right M14671
	left M14672
	unsp M14679
-	**Foot contractures**
	right M24574
	left M24575
	unsp M24576
-	**Foot crepitus (joint)**
	right M24174 left M24175 unsp M24176
M21379	**Foot drop acquired unsp**
	right M21371 left M21372
R601	**Foot edema NOS**
-	**Foot effusion**
	right M25474
	left M25475
	unsp M25476
-	**Foot fracture pathological NOS / (in neoplastic disease below)**
	unsp M84476- right M84474- left M84475-
	7th character indicates encounter/status
	A - initial S - sequela
	D - subsequent routine healing
	G - subsequent delayed healing
	K - subsequent nonunion P - subsequent malunion
	Change 4th character to 5 for 'in neoplastic disease'
	For fracture w/osteoporosis, see Foot osteoporosis
-	**Foot gout acute/NOS (and ankle)**
	idiopathic/primary right M10071 left M10072 unsp M10079
	lead induced right M10171 left M10172 unsp M10179
	drug induced right M10271 left M10272 unsp M10279
	d/t renal impairment right M10371 left M10372 unsp M10379
	other secondary right M10471 left M10472 unsp M10479

-	**Foot gout chronic (also ankle, toe)**
	idiopathic/primary right M1A071- left M1A072- unsp M1A079-
	lead induced right M1A171- left M1A172- unsp M1A179-
	drug induced right M1A271- left M1A272- unsp M1A279-
	d/t renal impairment right M1A371- left M1A372- unsp M1A379-
	other secondary right M1A471- left M1A472- unsp M1A479-
	The appropriate 7th character
	0 = without tophus (tophi) 1 = with tophus (tophi)
M25076	**Foot hemarthrosis unsp**
	right M25074 left M25075
M9279	**Foot joints chondromalacia unsp**
	right M94271 left M94272
-	**Foot mid-foot ulcer non-pressure chronic SEE HEEL**
M19079	**Foot osteoarthritis (& ankle) primary unsp**
	right M19071 left M19072
-	**Foot osteomyelitis NOS**
	acute hematogenous: right M86071 left M86072 unsp M86079
	acute other: right M86171 left M86172 unsp M86179
	subacute: right M86271 left M86272 unsp M86279
	chronic multifocal: right M86371 left M86372 unsp M86379
	chronic draining: right M86471 left M86472 unsp M86479
	chronic hematogenous: right M86571 left M86572 unsp M86579
	chronic other: right M86671 left M86672 unsp M86679
-	**Foot osteonecrosis**
	idiopathic: right M87074 left M87075 unsp M87076
	d/t drugs: right M87174 left M87175 unsp M87176
	d/t trauma: right M87274 left M87275 unsp M87276
	other secondary: right M87374 left M87375 unsp M87376
	other: right M87874 left M87875 unsp M87876
M80079-	**Foot osteoporosis age related w/current fracture unsp**
	right M80071- left M80072-
	7th character indicates encounter/status
	A - initial D - subsequent routine healing
	G - subsequent delayed healing S - sequela
	K - subsequent nonunion P - subsequent malunion
M25579	**Foot pain unsp**
	right M25571 left M25572
-	**Foot tendon rupture NOS non-traumatic / spontaneous**
	extensor: right M66271 left M66272 unsp M66279
	flexor: right M66371 left M66372 unsp M66379
	other: right M66871 left M66872 unsp M66879
L97429	**Foot ulcer non-pressure chronic left NOS**
	midfoot & heel:
	limited to skin: L97421
	fat layer exposed: L97422
	muscle necrosis: L97423
	bone necrosis: L97424
	Other part of foot - change 4th character to 5

L97419	**Foot ulcer non-pressure chronic right NOS**
	midfoot & heel --
	limited to skin L97411
	w/fat layer exposed L97412
	w/muscle necrosis L97413
	w/bone necrosis L97414
	Other part of foot - change 4th character to 5
L97409	**Foot ulcer non-pressure chronic unspec side NOS**
	midfoot & heel --
	limited to skin L97401
	w/fat layer exposed L97402
	w/muscle necrosis L97403
	w/bone necrosis L97404
	Other part of foot - change 4th character to 5
R627	**FTT: failure to thrive adult**
R509	**FUO: fever of unknown origin NOS**
D550	**G-6-PD: anemia/deficiency of G-6-PD**
F411	**GAD: generalized anxiety disorder**
K810	**Gallbladder abscess/empyema/gangrene NOS**
-	**Gallbladder calculus and bile duct calculus w/cholecystitis**
	NOS: K8060 w/obstruction K8061
	acute cholecystitis: K8062 w/obstruction K8063
	w/chronic cholecystitis: K8064 w/obstruction K8065
	w/acute & chronic cholecystitis: K8066 w/obstruction K8067
K824	**Gallbladder cholesterolosis / strawberry**
K829	**Gallbladder disease NOS**
	Also use for adhesions / atrophy / cyst / hypertrophy / ulcer
K823	**Gallbladder fistula**
K821	**Gallbladder hydrops / mucocele**
K820	**Gallbladder obstruction/occlusion/stenosis w/o cholelithiasis**
K822	**Gallbladder perforation**
K563	**Gallstone ileus**
K8020	**Gallstone impacted / NOS**
	impacted w/obstruction K8021
I96	**Gangrene cutaneous/ dry/ extremities/ moist/ spreading**
	gas A480
	presenile I731
	pulmonary J850
	Type 2 diabetes w/diabetic gangrene E1152
R141	**Gas pain**
B950	**GAS: group A streptococcal disease (as cause of other disease)**
K314	**Gastric diverticulum**
K316	**Gastric duodenal fistula**
K30	**Gastric hyperacidity**
K3189	**Gastric mucosa intestinal metaplasia**
K2960	**Gastric mucosal hypertrophy**
	w/ bleeding K2961
K311	**Gastric outlet obstruction**
K317	**Gastric polyp**

K3189	**Gastric prolapse/rupture**
K219	**Gastric reflux**
K259	**Gastric ulcer NOS**

        acute: w/hemorrhage K250 w/perforation K251
        acute: NOS K253 w/both hemorrhage/perforation K252
        chronic/unsp: w/hemorrhage K254 w/perforation K255
        chronic/unsp w/both hemorrhage/perforation K256
        chronic NOS K257

F458	**Gastritis nervous/psychogenic**
K2970	**Gastritis NOS**

        w/hemorrhage K2971
        acute: K2900   w/hemorrhage K2901
        alcoholic: K2920   w/hemorrhage K2921
        chronic: K2950   w/hemorrhage K2951
        chronic atrophic: K2940   w/hemorrhage K2941
        chronic superficial: K2930   w/hemorrhage K2931
        other: K2960   other w/hemorrhage K2961

K2990	**Gastroduodenitis NOS**

        w/bleeding K2991

K520	**Gastroenteritis d/t radiation**
K529	**Gastroenteritis non-infective NOS**

        granulomatous/regional/transmural K5010 (Crohn's)
        drug induced / toxic K521 code agent first
        allergic/dietetic K522   d/t radiation K520
        adaptive/membranous/mucous K589
        eosinophilic K5282

Z4659	**Gastrointestinal appliance fitting & adjustment**
K922	**Gastrointestinal bleeding/hemorrhage NOS**
K9281	**Gastrointestinal mucositis ulcerative**
K289	**Gastrojejunal ulcer NOS**

        acute: w/hemorrhage K280 w/perforation K281
        acute: NOS K283 w/both hemorrhage/perforation K282
        chronic/unsp: w/hemorrhage K284 w/perforation K285
        chronic/unsp w/both hemorrhage/perforation K286
        chronic NOS K287

K3184	**Gastroparesis**
Z431	**Gastrostomy care / aftercare**

        status w/o need for care Z931
        fitting & adjust Z4659

K9420	**Gastrostomy complication NOS**

        hemorrhage K9421   other K9429
        malfunction K9423   infection K9422
        for infection also code type
        eg. abd wall cellulitis L03.311 or a sepsis

B951	**GBS: group B streptococcal disease (as cause of other disease)**
G610	**GBS: Guillain-Barre' Syndrome**
O24419	**GDM: gestational diabetes mellitus NOS**

        diet controlled O24410

-	**Genital herpes SEE Herpes simplex Anogenital**

L293	**Genital itch**
N819	**Genital prolapse female unsp**
	uterovaginal: NOS N814 complete N813 incomplete N812
	urethrocele N810 rectocele N816
	cystocele: NOS N8110 lateral N8112 midline N8111
	vaginal enterocele N815 perineocele N8181
	cervical stump N8185 pelvic muscle wasting N8184
	incompetence of pubocervical tissue N8182
	incompetence of rectovaginal tissue N8183
	other N8189
T8351X-	**Genitourinary catheter infection**
	7th character indicates encounter
	A - initial encounter D - subsequent encounter S - sequela
K219	**GERD: gastroesophageal reflux disease**
	w/esophagitis K210
A071	**Giardiasis**
H44519	**Glaucoma absolute**
	right H44511 left H44512 bilateral H44513
-	**Glaucoma secondary to drugs (and selected others)**
	unsp eye H4060x- bilateral H4063x-
	right eye H4061x- left eye H4062x-
	If specified as secondary to eye inflammatiion 4th character = 4
	If specified as secondary to other eye disorder 4th character = 5
	if specified d/t trauma 4th character = 3
	0 - stage unspecified 1 - mild stage 2 - moderate stage
	3 - severe stage 4 - indeterminate stage
R7309	**Glucose abnormal NOS**
	aka latent diabetes, prediabetes
R7301	**Glucose fasting elevated/impaired**
R7302	**Glucose tolerance elevated/impaired (oral)**
E7400	**Glycogen storage disease NOS**
	type 1 E7401 type 2 E7402
	type 3 E7403 type 5 E7404
	other E7409
	RELATED cardiomyopathy I43
E012	**Goiter iodine deficiency NOS / endemic NOS**
	diffuse E010 multinodular E011
E049	**Goiter NOS**
	cystic NOS / nontoxic multinodular E042
	nontoxic uninodular E041
	nontoxic diffuse/simple E040
	toxic nodular E0520 w/crisis E0521
	iodine deficiency diffuse E010
	iodine deficiency multinodular E011
	iodine deficiency unsp E012
	dyshormogenetic E071
I43	**Gout cardiomyopathy**
M100	**Gout NOS**
	SEE Gout at foot, hand, hip, knee, elbow, toe, shoulder, wrist

M3130	**Granulomatosis respiratory necrotizing NOS**	
	w/renal involvement M3131	
E0500	**Grave's disease NOS**	
	w/ crisis E0501	
A8182	**GSS: Gerstmann-Straussler-Scheinker syndrome**	
R7309	**GTT: glucose tolerance test oral abnormal results (non-fasting)**	
G610	**Guillain-Barre syndrome**	
	also code sequelae G650	
-	**H&M: hematemesis and melena**	
	hematemesis K920 melena K921	
-	**Hallux disorders**	
	varus acquired unsp M2030 right M2031 left M2032	
	malleus acquired unsp M2040 right M2041 left M2042	
	rigidus acquired unsp M2020 right M2021 left M2022	
	valgus acquired unsp M2010 right M2011 left M2012	
-	**Hand bone cyst**	
	solitary cyst: unsp M85449 right M85441 left M85442	
	aneurysmal cyst: change 4th digit to 5	
	other cyst: change 4th digit to 6	
M7010	**Hand bursitis unsp**	
	right M7011 left M7012	
M71449	**Hand calcification unsp**	
	right M71441 left M71442	
M9249	**Hand chondromalacia unsp**	
	right M94241 left M94242	
-	**Hand fracture pathological NOS / (in neoplastic disease below)**	
	unsp M84443- right M84441- left M84442-	
	7th character indicates encounter/status	
	A - initial S - sequela	
	D - subsequent routine healing	
	G - subsequent delayed healing	
	K - subsequent nonunion P - subsequent malunion	
	Change 4th character to 5 for 'in neoplastic disease'	
-	**Hand gout acute / NOS**	
	idiopathic/primary right M10041 left M10042 unsp M10049	
	drug induced right M10241 left M10242 unsp M10249	
	d/t renal impairment right M10341 left M10342 unsp M10349	
	lead induced right M10141 left M10142 unsp M10149	
	other secondary right M10441 left M10442 unsp M10449	
-	**Hand gout chronic**	
	idiopathic/primary right M1A041- left M1A042- unsp M1A049-	
	lead induced right M1A141- left M1A142- unsp M1A149-	
	drug induced right M1A241- left M1A242- unsp M1A249-	
	d/t renal impairment right M1A341- left M1A342- unsp M1A349-	
	other secondary right M1A441- left M1A442- unsp M1A449-	
	The appropriate 7th character	
	0 = without tophus (tophi) 1 = with tophus (tophi)	
M25049	**Hand hemarthrosis unsp**	
	right M25041 left M25042	

M19049	**Hand osteoarthritis primary unsp**
	right M19041 left M19042
M80049-	**Hand osteoporosis age related w/current fracture unsp**
	right M80041- left M80042-
	7th character indicates encounter/status
	A - initial D - subsequent routine healing
	G - subsequent delayed healing S - sequela
	K - subsequent nonunion P - subsequent malunion
G4732	**HAPB: high altitude periodic breathing**
I119	**HCVD: hypertensive cardiovascular disease NOS**
	w/heart failure I110
G44009	**Headache Cluster NOS**
	intractable G44001
	episodic: NOS G44019 intractable G44011
	chronic: NOS G44029 intractable G44021
G4440	**Headache drug induced NEC NOS**
	intractable G4441
R51	**Headache NOS SEE migraine if specified**
-	**Headache other specified**
	primary thunderclap G4453
	hypnic G4481
	primary cough G4483
	primary exertional G4484
	primary stabbing G4485
	new daily persistent G4452
G44309	**Headache Post-traumatic NOS**
	NOS intractable G44301
	acute: NOS G44319 intractale G44311
	chronic: NOS G44329 intractable G44321
G43C0	**Headache syndrome periodic NOS**
	intractable G43C1
G44209	**Headache Tension NOS**
	intractable G44201
	episodic: NOS G44219 intractable G44211
	chronic: NOS G44229 intractable G44221
G441	**Headache vascular NEC**
I447	**Heart block left bundle branch NOS**
	left bundle branch hemi NOS I4460
	left anterior fascicular I444
	left posterior fascicular I445
I459	**Heart block NOS**
	bundle branch NOS I454 sinoatrial I455
	bifascicular I452 trifascicular I453
	AV NOS I4430 AV other I4439
	AV 1st degree I440 AV 2nd degree I441
	AV 3rd degree / complete I442
I4510	**Heart block right bundle branch NOS**
	right fascicular I450
	right other I4519

I119	**Heart disease hypertensive NOS**
	w/heart failure I110 also code heart failure
-	**Heart disease hypertensive w/ chronic kidney disease**
	w/o heart failure -
	w/ CKD stages 1-4 or unsp I1310
	w/CKD stage 5 (ESRD) I1311
	w/heart failure -
	w/CKD stages 1-4 or unsp I130
	w/CKD stage 5 (ESRD) I132
	RELATED Chronic kidney disease
	stage 1 N181 stage 2 N182
	stage 3 N183 stage 4 N184
	stage 5 N185 end stage N186
I259	**Heart disease ischemic chronic/NOS**
-	**Heart disease rheumatic acute**
	pericarditis I010 endocarditis I011
	myocarditis I012 other spec I018
	unsp / carditis I019
I069	**Heart disease rheumatic chronic AORTIC VALVE unsp**
	stenosis I060 insufficiency I061
	stenosis w/insufficiency I062
	other specified I068
I059	**Heart disease rheumatic chronic MITRAL VALVE unsp**
	stenosis I050 insufficiency I051
	stenosis w/insufficiency I052
	other specified I058
I089	**Heart disease rheumatic chronic MULTIPLE VALVE unsp**
	mitral & aortic NOS I080
	mitral & triscupid NOS I081
	aortic & tricuspid NOS I082
	mitral & aortic & tricuspid NOS I083
	other NOS I088
I079	**Heart disease rheumatic chronic TRICUSPID VALVE unsp**
	stenosis I070 insufficiency I071
	stenosis w/insufficiency I072
	other specified I078
I099	**Heart disease rheumatic unsp**
	myocarditis I090
	endocarditis I091
	chronic pericarditis I092
	heart failure I0981
	other specified I0989
I499	**Heart dysrhythmia NOS**
I517	**Heart enlarged**

I509	**Heart failure congestive NOS**
	systolic: acute I5021 chronic I5022
	systolic: acute on chronic I5023 unsp I5020
	diastolic: acute I5031 chronic I5032
	diastolic: acute on chronic I5033 unsp I5030
	combined systolic-diastolic:
	acute I5041 chronic I5042
	acute on chronic I5043 unsp I5040
I509	**Heart failure NOS**
-	**Heart failure postop (code before type of failure)**
	cardiac surgery I97130
	other surgery I97131
R002	**Heart palpitations**
-	**Heart valve disorders nonrheumatic**
	PULMONARY unsp I379 other I378 stenosis I370
	insufficiency I371 stenosis w/insufficiency I372
	TRICUSPID unsp I369 other I368 stenosis I360
	insufficiency I361 stenosis w/insufficiency I362
	AORTIC unsp I359 other I358 stenosis I350
	insufficiency I351 stenosis w/insufficiency I352
	MITRAL unsp I349 other I348 stenosis I340
	insufficiency I341 stenosis w/insufficiency I342
R12	**Heartburn**
L97429	**Heel ulcer non-pressure chronic left NOS**
	limited to skin: L97421
	fat layer exposed: L97422
	muscle necrosis: L97423
	bone necrosis: L97424
L97419	**Heel ulcer non-pressure chronic right NOS**
	limited to skin L97411
	w/fat layer exposed L97412
	w/muscle necrosis L97413
	w/bone necrosis L97414
L97409	**Heel ulcer non-pressure chronic unspec side NOS**
	limited to skin L97401
	w/fat layer exposed L97402
	w/muscle necrosis L97403
	w/bone necrosis L97404
L89629	**Heel ulcer pressure left NOS**
	unstageable L89620
	stage 1 L89621 stage 2 L89622
	stage 3 L89623 stage 4 L89624
L89619	**Heel ulcer pressure right NOS**
	unstageable L89610
	stage 1 L89611 stage 2 L89612
	stage 3 L89613 stage 4 L89614

L89609	**Heel ulcer pressure unspecified side NOS**
	unstageable L89600
	stage 1 L89601 stage 2 L89602
	stage 3 L89603 stage 4 L89604
M2500	**Hemarthrosis NOS**
K920	**Hematemesis**
K921	**Hematochezia**
R710	**Hematocrit precipitous drop (or hemoglobin)**
M7981	**Hematoma soft tissue nontraumatic**
	SEE Postop also
N857	**Hematometra**
N836	**Hematosalpinx**
	w/hematometra N857
R319	**Hematuria NOS**
	gross R310
	benign essential microscopic R311
	other microscopic R312
	SEE cystitis or other condition for combined codes
N029	**Hematuria recurrent and persistent**
	w/minor glomerular abnormality N020
	w/focal & segmental glomerular lesions N021
	w/diffuse membranous glomerulonephritis N022
	w/diffuse mesangial proliferative glomerulonephritis N023
	w/diffuse endocapillary proliferative glomerulonephritis N024
	w/diffuse mesangiocapillary glomerulonephritis N025
	w/dense deposit disease N026
	w/diffuse crescentic glomerulonephritis N027
	w/other morphologic changes N028
G8100	**Hemiplegia & hemiparesis Flaccid NOS**
	dominant side right G8101 left G8102
	nondominant right G8103 left G8104
G8190	**Hemiplegia & hemiparesis NOS**
	dominant side right G8191 left G8192
	nondominant right G8193 left G8194
G8110	**Hemiplegia & hemiparesis Spastic**
	dominant side right G8111 left G8112
	nondominant right G8113 left G8114
E83119	**Hemochromatosis unsp**
	d/t repeated red blood cell tranfusions E83111
	hereditary E83110
	other E83118
D66	**Hemophilia NOS / A**
	hemophilia B D67
	hemophilia C D681
	vascular D680
R042	**Hemoptysis**
D6832	**Hemorrhage anticoagulant induced**
N950	**Hemorrhage postmenopausal**

K649	**Hemorrhoids NOS (bleeding)**
	stage 1 K640 bleed w/o prolapse
	stage 2 K641 bleed/ prolapse w/strain, then retract
	stage 3 K642 bleed/ prolapse, require manual replace
	stage 4 K643 bleed/ prolapse, cannot replace manually
	external NOS/ perianal venous thrombosis K644
	external thrombosed K645
	other K648
-	**Hepatic - SEE also Liver**
K7291	**Hepatic coma NOS**
K7010	**Hepatitis alcoholic NOS**
	w/ascites K7011
K754	**Hepatitis autoimmune / Lupoid NEC**
K753	**Hepatitis granulomatous NEC**
K752	**Hepatitis nonspecific reactive**
B159	**Hepatitis viral acute A NOS**
	w/hepatic coma B150
B169	**Hepatitis viral acute B NOS**
	NOS w/delta agent B161
	w/delta agent w/hepatic coma B160
	w/hepatic coma B162
B179	**Hepatitis viral acute NOS**
	acute delta super infectiion of B carrier B170
	hepatitis C NOS B1710
	hepatits C w/hepatic coma B1711
	hepatitis E acute B172
	other specified NEC B178
B189	**Hepatitis viral chronic NOS**
	hepatitis NOS B B181 w/delta agent B180
	hepatitis C B182
	other chronic B188
B942	**Hepatitis viral SEQUELAE**
B199	**Hepatitis viral unspecified NOS**
	NOS w/coma B190
	B NOS B1910 B NOS w/coma B1911
	C NOS B1920 C NOS w/coma B1921
A609	**Herpes simplex infection ANOGENITAL NOS**
	penis A6001 other male genital A6002
	cervicitis A6003
	vulvovaginitis / vulva / vagina A6004
	other urogenital tract A6009
	perianal skin and rectum A601

B009	**Herpes simplex infection NOS**
	eczema herpeticum B000 meningitis B003
	vesicular dermatitis B001 encephalitis B004
	gingivostomatitis /pharyngitis B002
	disseminated /sepsis B007
	hepatitis B0081 myelitis B0082
	other/ whitlow B0089
	ocular NOS B0050 iridocyclitis/ uveitis B0051
	keratitis B0052 conjunctivitis B0053
	other ocular B0059
B0082	**Herpes simplex RELATED Myelitis**
B029	**Herpes zoster NOS**
	w/myelitis B0224 polyneuropathy B0223
	geniculate B0221 conjunctivitis B0231
	iridocyclitis B0232 scleritis B0234
	keratoconjunctivitis B0233 meningitis B021
	opthalmicus B0239 encephalitis B020
	disseminated B027 w/other complications B028
B084	**HFMD: hand foot mouth disease**
E791	**HG-PRT: hypoxanthine-guanine-phosphoribosyl transferase deficiency**
-	**HGSIL: high grade squamous intraepithelial lesion**
	from vaginal pap smear: R87623
	from cervix pap smear: R87613
Q871	**HHHO: hypotonia, hypomentia, hypogonadism, obesity syndrome**
K449	**Hiatel hernia NOS**
	incarcerated/ irreducible/ obstructive/ strangulated K440
	w/gangrene K441
-	**Hip abrasion NOS**
	right S70211- left S70212- unsp S70219
	7th character indicates encounter
	A - initial encounter D - subsequent encounter S - sequela
M24659	**Hip ankylosis unsp**
	right M24651 left M24652
-	**Hip arthritis NOS**
	allergic/ climacteric: unsp M13859 right M13851 left M13852
	crystal NOS: unsp M11859 right M11851 left M11852
	degenerative: SEE hip osteoarthritis
	transient: unsp M12859 right M12851 left M12852
	traumatic: unsp M12559 right M12551 left M12552
M25759	**Hip bone spur (osteophyte) unsp**
	right M25751 left M25752
-	**Hip bursitis**
	trochanteric unsp M7060 right M7061 left M7062
	other unsp M7070 right M7071 left J7072
M71459	**Hip calcification unsp**
	right M71451 left M71452
M9259	**Hip chondromalacia unsp**
	right M94251 left M94252

M24559	**Hip contractures unsp**
	right M24551 left M24552
-	**Hip dislocation**

        NOS: unsp S73006-   right NOS S73004-   left NOS S73005-
        posterior: unsp S73016-   right S73014-   left S73015-
        central: unsp S73046-   right S73044-   left S73045-
        obturator: unsp S73026-   right S73024-   left S73025-
        other anterior: NOS S73036-   right S73034-   left S73035-
        7th character indicates encounter
        A - initial encounter D - subsequent encounter S - sequela

M24459	**Hip dislocation recurrent unsp**
	right M24451 left M24452
-	**Hip fixation internal infected**

        right T84620-   left T84621-
        7th character indicates encounter
        A - initial encounter D - subsequent encounter S - sequela

- **Hip fracture closed NOS**

        right S72001-   Left S72002-   unsp S72009-
        7th character indicates encounter/status
        A - initial
        D - subsequent routine healing
        G - subsequent delayed healing
        K - subsequent nonunion
        P - subsequent malunion
        S - sequela

M84459   **Hip fracture pathological NOS / (in neoplastic disease below)**

        femur: unsp M84453-   right M84451-   left M84452-
        7th character indicates encounter/status
        A - initial   S - sequela
        D - subsequent routine healing
        G - subsequent delayed healing
        K - subsequent nonunion   P - subsequent malunion
        Change 4th character to 5 for 'in neoplastic disease'

- **Hip gout acute/NOS**

        idiopathic/primary right M10051 left M10052   unsp M10059
        lead induced right M10151   left M10152   unsp M10159
        drug induced right M10251 left M10252   unsp M10259
        d/t renal impairment right M10351   left M10352 unsp M10359
        other secondary right M10451 left M10452   unsp M10459

- **Hip gout chronic**

        idiopathic/primary right M1A051- left M1A052-   unsp M1A059-
        lead induced right M1A151-   left M1A152-   unsp M1A159-
        drug induced right M1A251- left M1A252-   unsp M1A259-
        d/t renal impairment right M1A351-   left M1A352- unsp M1A359-
        other secondary right M1A451- left M1A452-   unsp M1A459-
        The appropriate 7th character
        0 = without tophus (tophi)   1 = with tophus (tophi)

M25059   **Hip hemarthrosis unsp**

        right M25051   left M25052

-	**Hip injuries superficial**

        Contusion
        unsp S70.00x-   right S70.01x-   left S70.02x-
        Abrasion
        unsp S70219-   right S70211-   left S70212-
        Blister (nonthermal)
        unsp S70221-   right S70222-   left S70229-
        Insect bite (nonvenomous)
        unsp S70269-   right S70261-   left S70262-
        7th character indicates encounter
        A - initial encounter D - subsequent encounter S - sequela

M24859   **Hip joint instability NOS unsp**
        right M4851   left M24852

M24059   **Hip joint mice unsp**
        right M24051   left M24052

-   **Hip joint prosthetic complication mechanical RIGHT**
        broken T84010-
        dislocation T84020-
        mechanical loosening T84030-
        peri prosthetic: fracture T84042- osteolysis T84050-
        wear of articular bearing surface T84060-
        7th character indicates encounter
        A - initial encounter D - subsequent encounter S - sequela
        Change 6th character for LEFT hip joint = 1

M169   **Hip osteoarthritis NOS**
        Primary: bilateral M160   unsp M1610
        Primary: right M1611   left M1612
        d/t dysplasia: bilateral M162 unsp M1630
        d/t dysplasia: right M1631   left M1632
        post trauma: bilateral M164 unsp M1650
        post trauma: right M1651   left M1652
        other bilateral: M166   other unilateral: M167

M87059   **Hip osteonecrosis idiopathic aseptic NOS**

M80059   **Hip osteoporosis w/current pathological fracture unsp**
        right M80051   left M80052
        7th character indicates encounter/status
        A - initial
        D - subsequent routine healing
        G - subsequent delayed healing
        K - subsequent nonunion
        P - subsequent malunion
        S - sequela

M25559   **Hip pain unsp**
        right M25551   left M25552

L89229   **Hip pressure ulcer left NOS**
        unstageable L89220
        stage 1 L89221   stage 2 L89222
        stage 3 L89223   stage 4 L89224

L89219	**Hip pressure ulcer right NOS**
	unstageable L89210
	stage 1 L89211 stage 2 L89212
	stage 3 L89213 stage 4 L89214
L89209	**Hip pressure ulcer unspecified side NOS**
	unstageable L89200
	stage 1 L89201 stage 2 L89202
	stage 3 L89203 stage 4 L89204
Z96649	**Hip replacement status NOS**
	right Z96641 left Z96642 bilat Z96643
D7582	**HIT: heparin induced thrombocytopenia**
B9735	**HIV 2: human immunodeficiency virus type 2 infection**
	used as cause of other disease
Z717	**HIV counseling**
Z21	**HIV infection asymptomatic status**
R75	**HIV serologic evidence inconclusive**
B20	**HIV: human immunodeficiency virus infection NOS**
L509	**Hives NOS**
M5030	**HNP: herniated nucleus palposus cervical NOS**
M5136	**HNP: herniated nucleus palposus lumbar**
M5134	**HNP: herniated nucleus palposus thoracic**
D751	**HOA: high oxygen affinity hemoglobin polycythemia**
	secondary polycythemia
-	**Hodgkin lymphoma (lymph nodes)**
	Nodular lymphocyte predominant type:
	unsp nodes C8100 head/face/neck C8101 intrathoracic C8102
	intra-abdominal C8103 axilla / arm C8104 inguinal / leg C8105
	intrapelvic C8106 spleen C8107 multiple C8108 extranodal C8109
	For other type Hodgkin, change 4th character
	1 = Nodular sclerosis classical 2 = Mixed cellularity classical
	3 = Lymphocyte depleted classical
	4 = Lymphocyte rich classical 7 = other classical
	9 = unspecified
	Personal hx of Hodgkin lymphoma Z8571
H9190	**HOH: hard of hearing unsp**
	right ear H9191 left ear H9192 bilateral H9193
	used to code deaf NOS
B769	**Hookworm NOS**
	ancylostomiasis B760
	necatoriasis B761
	other B768
Z79890	**Hormone replacement therapy postmenopausal**
Z515	**Hospice care (terminal care/ palliative care)**
M8940	**HPOA: hypertrophic pulmonary osteoarthropathy NOS**
Z1151	**HPV screening: human papilloma virus screening**
A630	**HPV: human papillomavirus infection (anogenital warts)**
Z79890	**HRT: hormone replacement therapy (postmenopausal) long term**
R162	**HSM: hepatosplenomegaly NOS**
B0082	**HSM: herpes simplex myelitis**

B003	**HSM: herpex simplex meningitis**
D690	**HSP: Henoch-Schonlein purpura (allergic)**
B009	**HSV: herpes simplex virus infection NOS**
B9733	**HTLV-I: human T-cell lymphotrophic virus type I cause of other disease** HTLV-II B9734
I10	**HTN: hypertension NOS includes high blood pressure, essential, primary, benign, malignant**
-	**HTR: hemolytic transfusion reaction** acute d/t Rh incompatibility T80410- acute d/t ABO incompatibility T80310- delayed 24 hr+ d/t Rh incompatibility T80411- delayed 24 hr+ d/t ABO incompatibility T80311- unsp d/t Rh incompatibility T80419- unsp d/t ABO incompatibility T80319- 7th character indicates encounter A - initial encounter D - subsequent encounter S - sequela
E8381	**Hungry bone syndrome**
G10	**Huntington's chorea**
D593	**HUS: hemolytic uremic syndrome** RELATED pneumococcal pneumonia J13 RELATED shigella dyenteriae A039 RELATED e colli infection B962- final character below NOS 0 STEC 0157 1 other spec STEC 2 other unsp STEC 3 non STEC 9
N433	**Hydrocele of spermatic cord, testis or tunica vaginalis unsp** encysted N430 infected N431 other N432
G919	**Hydrocephalus NOS** communicating G910 obstructive G911 normal pressure G912 post trauma NOS G913 in other disease G914 code other disease first other G918
N1330	**Hydronephrosis NOS** w/ureteral stricture NEC N131 w/ renal & ureteral calculous obstruction N132 infected N136 other N1339
N134	**Hydroureter NOS** infected N136
E269	**Hyperaldosteronism NOS (also aldosteronism)** other primary E2609 Secondary E261 Bartler's E2681 Conn's syndrome E2601 glucocorticoid-remediable E2602
E8352	**Hypercalcemia**
R739	**Hyperglycemia NOS** post-pancreatectomy E891

E781	**Hyperglyceridemia endogenous/pure**
	mixed E783
	w/hypercholesterolemia E782
E7251	**Hyperglycinemia non-ketotic**
E875	**Hyperkalemia**
E785	**Hyperlipidemia unsp**
M4810	**Hyperostosis ankylosing (diffuse idiopathic skeletal) NOS**
	occipito-atlanto-axial M4811
	cervical M4812
	cervicothoracic M4813
	thoracic M4814
	thoracolumbar M4815
	lumbar M4816
	lumbosacral M4817
	sacral and sacrococcygeal M4818
	multiple sites M4819
E213	**Hyperparathyroidism NOS**
	primary E210
	secondary / NEC E211
	secondary of renal origin N2581
	other E212 ectopic E342
D731	**Hypersplenism**
I10	**Hypertension essential/primary**
	RELATED exp to environmental smoke occupational Z5731
	RELATED exp to environmental smoke NOS Z7722
	RELATED hx of tobacco use Z87891 tobacco use Z720
K766	**Hypertension portal**
	RELATED gastropathy K3189
I272	**Hypertension pulmonary NOS**
	pulmonary primary I270
I159	**Hypertension secondary NOS**
	renovascular I150 d/t other renal disorders I151
	d/t endocrine disorders I152 other I158
	postop I973
E8351	**Hypocalcemia**
E162	**Hypoglycemia NOS**
	diabetic: NOS E11649 w/coma E11641
	nondiabetic drug induced: NOS E160 w/coma E15
	other nondiabetic E161
E876	**Hypokalemia**
	RELATED nephropathy from impaired renal function N2589
E209	**Hypoparathyroidism NOS**
	idiopathic E200 pseudo E201
	other E208
	postop E892

I959	**Hypotension NOS**
	idiopathic I950 d/t drugs I952
	d/t hemodialysis I953
	orthostatic/postural I951
	postpro I9581
	chronic/(permanent idiopathic) / other I9589
	cardiovascular collapse (shock) R579
	nonspecific low blood pressure reading NOS R031
	neurogenic orthostatic (Shy-Drager) G903
E039	**Hypothyroidism NOS/primary**
	d/t iodine / PAS/ iatrogenic E032
	secondary acquired NOS E038
	postop or d/t radiation therapy E890
	congenital E009
	postinfectious E033
E861	**Hypovolemia**
B0224	**HZM: herpes zoster myelitis**
K5090	**IBD: inflammatory bowel disease NOS**
	SEE Crohn's disease unspecified intestine for more
G7241	**IBM: inclusion body myositis**
K589	**IBS: irritable bowel syndrome**
	w/ diarrhea K580
N3010	**IC: interstitial cystitis chronic (or ICC)**
	with hematuria N3011
F79	**ID: intellectual disability NOS**
	mild IQ 50-70 F70
	moderate IQ 35-55 F71
	severe IQ 20-40 F72
	profound IQ below 20 F73
	other F78
H2181	**IFIS: intraoperative floppy iris syndrome**
E269	**IHA: idiopathic hyperaldosteronism**
I259	**IHD: ischemic heart disease NOS (chronic)**
I421	**IHSS: idiopathic hypertrophic subaortic stenosis**
K529	**Ileitis NOS noninfective**
	regional K5000 (Crohn's)
K632	**Ileorectal fistula**
Z432	**Ileostomy care / aftercare**
	status w/o need for care Z932
K9410	**Ileostomy complication NOS**
	hemorrhage K9411 malfunction K9413
	other K9419 infection K9412
	for infection also code type eg. abd wall cellulitis L03311 or a sepsis
	granulation of surrounding skin L928
K560	**Ileus paralytic/(secondary NOS) of colon or small intestine**
	gallstone ileus K563
	unsp ileus K567
I723	**Iliac artery aneurysm**
I7772	**Iliac artery dissection**

D819	**Immunodeficiency severe combined NOS**
	w/ reticular dysgenesis D810
	w/ low T and B cell numbers D811
	ww/ low or normal B cell numbers D812
H6120	**Impaction cerumen NOS**
	right ear H6121 left H6122
	bilat H6123
L0100	**Impetigo NOS**
	Non-bullous L0101
	Brockhart's/follicularis L0102
	Bullous/neonatorum L0103
	Other/ulcerative L0109
E46	**Inanition NOS**
	w/edema E43
	d/t food deprivation T730XX-
	7th character indicates encounter
	A - initial encounter D - subsequent encounter S - sequela
K432	**Incisional hernia ventral NOS**
	incarcerated K430
	gangrenous K431
K30	**Indigestion**
-	**INFECTION GENERALIZED -- SEE sepsis**
	For specific see site, type or source
Z1630	**Infection resistant to drug - unspecifed**
	ampicillin / penicillin Z1611
	sulfonamides/ tetracylines / Kanomycin/ Streptomycin Z1629
	cephalosporins Z1610 multiple drugs unspec Z1624
	quinolones/fluoroquinolones Z1623
	Vancomycin Z1621 Vancomycin related Z1622
	antivirals Z1633 antifungals Z1632
-	**Influenza & pneumonia RELATED codes**
	lung abscess w/pneumonia J851 w/o pneumonia J852
	pleural effusion in other conditions J918
	sinusitis unsp J0190 unsp recurrent J0191 SEE sinusitis for more
	tympanic membrane rupture NOS: unsp ear H7290
	right ear H7291 left ear H7292 bilat H7293
-	**Influenza d/t novel influenza A virus (avian, bird, swine, H5N1)**
	w/pneumonia J09x1
	w/other respiratory manifestations J09x2
	w/gastrointestinal manifestations J09x3
	w/other manifestations J09x9

-	**Influenza d/t other identified influenza virus**
	w/unspecified pneumonia J1000
	w/pneumonia d/t same virus J1001
	w/pneumonia d/t different virus J1008
	w/other respiratory manifestations J101
	w/gastrointestinal manifestations J102
	w/encephalopathy J1081 w/myocarditis J1082
	w/otitis media J1083
	w/other manifestations J1089
	RELATED pleural effusion J918 lung abscess J851
	acute sinusitis NOS J0190 see sinusitis for more
J111	**Influenza NOS (d/t unidentified virus)**
	w/gastrointestinal manifestations J112
	w/encephalopathy J1181
	w/myocarditis J1182
	w/otitis media J1183
	w/other manifestations J1189
Z451	**Infusion pump adjustment and management**
T8572x-	**Infusion pump site infected**
	7th character indicates encounter
	A - initial encounter D - subsequent encounter S - sequela
K4020	**Inguinal hernia bilateral NOS**
	recurrent K4021
	bilat: w/obstruction NOS K4000 recurrent K4001
	bilat: w/gangrene NOS K4010 recurrent K4011
K4090	**Inguinal hernia unilateral NOS - right or left code same**
	recurrent K4091
K4040	**Inguinal hernia unilateral w/ gangrene NOS - right or left code same**
	recurrent K4041
K4030	**Inguinal hernia unilateral w/obstruction NOS - right or left code same**
	recurrent K4031
I889	**Inguinal lymphadenitis NOS**
	acute L041 chronic I881
G912	**INPH: idiopathic normal pressure hydrocephalus**
	secondary INPH G910
G4700	**Insomnia NOS**
	d/t medical condition G4701 also code condition
	primary F5101
	d/t mental disorder F5105
	other NEC G4709
T383X5-	**Insulin adverse effect**
	7th character indicates encounter
	A - initial encounter D - subsequent encounter S - sequela
Z4681	**Insulin pump fitting & adjustment**

Z9641	**Insulin Pump presence**
	fit & adjust & training Z4681
	For T codes below, 7th character indicates encounter
	A - initial encounter D - subsequent encounter S - sequela
	mechanical breakdown T85614-
	displacement T85624- leakage T85633-
	infection/inflammation d/t T8572x-
-	**Insulin toxicity**
	accidental/NOS T383X1-
	adverse effect T383X5-
	underdosing T383X6-
	7th character indicates encounter
	A - initial encounter D - subsequent encounter S - sequela
Z4659	**Intestinal appliance fitting & adjustment**
K5660	**Intestinal obstruction NOS**
-	**Intestine small diverticular disease**
	diverticulitis w/perforation & abscess K5700
	diverticulitis w/perforation & abscess w/bleeding K5701
	diverticulitis: NOS K5712 w/bleeding K5713
	diverticulosis: NOS K5710 w/bleeding K5711
-	**Intestine small neoplasm SEE colon for large intestine**
	Malignant primary
	jejunum C171 benign D1339
	ileum C172 benign D1339
	Meckel's diverticulum C173
	overlapping sites C178
	unsp / NOS C179 benignD1330
	duodenum C170 benign D132
	Secondary (all) C784
	Mets to bone C7951 mets to unsp lymph nodes C779
	Mets to intraabdominal lymph node C772
K5660	**Intestine small obstruction NOS**
K631	**Intestine small perforation**
K614	**Intrasphincteric abscess / cellulitis**
E222	**ISADH: inappropriate secretion of antidiuretic hormone syndrome**
K613	**Ischiorectal abscess / cellulitis**
N3642	**ISD: intrinsic sphincter deficiency (urethral)**
	w/ urethral hypermobility N3643
A073	**Isosporiasis**
L299	**Itch NOS**
	genital unsp L293
	perianal L290 ani L290
	winter L298 scroti L291
	vulva L292
D693	**ITP: idiopathic thrombocytopenic purpura**
Z452	**IV catheter adjustment and management**

-	**IV caused infection**
	bloodstream infection T80211-
	local T80212-
	other T80218-
	unsp infection T80219-
	7th character indicates encounter
	A - initial encounter D - subsequent encounter S - sequela
-	**IVDP: interertebral disc prolapse NOD SEE HNP**
I615	**IVH: intraventricular hemorrhage adult (nontraumatic)**
Z4803	**Jackson Pratt post op drain change / removal**
M081	**JAS: juvenile ankylosing spondylitis**
R17	**Jaundice NOS / symptomatic**
-	**Joint mice SEE joint site**
-	**Joint prosthetic complication mechanical unsp joint**
	broken T84019-
	dislocation T84029-
	mechanical loosening T84039-
	peri prosthetic: fracture T84049- osteolysis T84059-
	wear of articular bearing surface T84069-
	7th character indicates encounter
	A - initial encounter D - subsequent encounter S - sequela
	Change 6th character for known joint:
	0 = right hip 1 = left hip 2 = right knee 3 = left knee 8 = other
M0800	**JRA: juvenile rheumatoid arthritis NOS**
C469	**Kaposi's sarcoma NOS**
	skin C460 soft tissue C461
	palate C462 lymph nodes C463
	gastrointestinal sites C464
	lung: unsp C4650 right C4651 left C4652
	other sites C467
L821	**Keratosis seborrheic NOS**
	inflamed L820
N151	**Kidney abscess/carbuncle/cellulitis**
N2889	**Kidney adhesions**
N261	**Kidney atrophy terminal**
N200	**Kidney calculus**
	w/calculus of ureter N202
N281	**Kidney cyst acquired**
I129	**Kidney disease chronic hypertensive NOS / stages 1-4 ckd**
	w/stage 5 ckd I120
	Also code ckd stage
N189	**Kidney disease chronic NOS**
	stage 1 N181 stage 2 mild N182
	stage 3 moderate N183 stage 4 severe N184
	stage 5 N185 end stage N186
	For stage 6 (and stage) also code dialysis status Z992
D631	**Kidney disease chronic RELATED anemia**
N2581	**Kidney disease RELATED hyperparathyroidism secondary**

N179	**Kidney failure acute NOS**
	w/tubular necrosis N170
	w/acute cortical necrosis N171
	w/medullary necrosis N172
	other N178
N19	**Kidney failure NOS**
N269	**Kidney fibrosis NOS**
N2889	**Kidney hemorrhage**
N2881	**Kidney hypertrophy**
N280	**Kidney ischemia / infarction**
N289	**Kidney lesion/mass**
-	**Kidney neoplasm except renal pelvis**
	MALIGNANT primary
	right C641 left C642 unsp C649
	Secondary unsp C7900 right C7901 left C7902
	Benign unsp D3000 right D3001 left D3002
	Mets to bone C7951 mets to unsp lymph nodes C779
	Mets to intraabdominal lymph node C772
-	**Kidney neoplasm renal pelvis**
	MALIGNANT primary
	right C651 left C652 unsp C659
	Secondary unsp C7900 right C7901 left C7902
	Benign unsp D3010 right D3011 left D3012
	Mets to bone C7951 mets to unsp lymph nodes C779
	Mets to intraabdominal lymph node C772
	Mets to intrapelvic lymph node C775
N269	**Kidney sclerosis NOS**
N279	**Kidney small NOS**
	unilateral N270 bilateral N271
N200	**Kidney stone**
	kidney stone w/ureter stone N202
M4820	**Kissing spine NOS**
	occipito-atlanto-axial M4821
	cervical M4822
	cervicothoracic M4823
	thoracic M4824
	thoracolumbar M4825
	lumbar M4826
	lumbosacral M4827
L03115	**Knee abscess NOS right**
	left L03116
M24669	**Knee ankylosis unsp**
	right M24661 left M24662
-	**Knee arthritis infectious**
	in other disease infective right M01x61 left M01x62 NOS M01x69
	pyogenic staph: right M00061 left M00062 unsp M00069
	pneumococcal: right M00161 left M00162 unsp M00169
	other strep: right M00261 left M00262 unsp M00269
	other bacteria: right M00861 left M00862 unsp M00869

-	**Knee bursitis NOS**	
	prepatellar: unsp M7040 right M7041 left M7042	
	other: unsp M7050 right M7051 left M7052	
M71469	**Knee calcification unsp**	
	right M71461 left M71462	
M2240	**Knee chondromalacia patellae unsp**	
	right M2241 left M2242	
M9269	**Knee chondromalacia unsp**	
	right M94261 left M94262	
M24569	**Knee contractures unsp**	
	right M24561 left M24562	
M25469	**Knee effusion (joint) unsp**	
	right 25461 left M25412	
-	**Knee gout acute/NOS**	
	idiopathic/primary: right M10061 left M10062 unsp M10069	
	lead induced: right M10161 left M10162 unsp M10169	
	drug induced: right M10261 left M10262 unsp M10269	
	d/t renal impairment: right M10361 left M10362 unsp M10369	
	other secondary: right M10461 left M10462 unsp M10469	
-	**Knee gout chronic**	
	idiopathic/primary right M1A061- left M1A062- unsp M1A069-	
	lead induced right M1A161- left M1A162- unsp M1A169-	
	drug induced right M1A261- left M1A262- unsp M1A269-	
	d/t renal impairment right M1A361- left M1A362- unsp M1A369-	
	other secondary right M1A461- left M1A462- unsp M1A469-	
	The appropriate 7th character	
	0 = without tophus (tophi) 1 = with tophus (tophi)	
M25069	**Knee hemarthrosis unsp**	
	right M25061 left M25062	
M2340	**Knee joint mice unsp**	
	right M2341 left M2342	
-	**Knee joint prosthetic complication mechanical RIGHT**	
	broken T84012-	
	instability T84022-	
	mechanical loosening T84032-	
	peri prosthetic: fracture T84042- osteolysis T84052-	
	wear of articular bearing surface T84062-	
	7th character indicates encounter	
	A - initial encounter D - subsequent encounter S - sequela	
	Change 6th character for LEFT knee joint = 3	
M179	**Knee osteoarthritis NOS**	
	primary: right M1711 left M1712 bilateral M170 unsp M1710	
	post-trauma: right M1731 left M1732 unsp M1730	
	other secondary unilateral M175	
	other secondary bilat M174	
M25569	**Knee pain unsp**	
	right M25561 left M25562	
Z96659	**Knee replacement status NOS**	
	right Z96651 left Z96652 bilat Z96653	

C469	**KS: Kaposi's sarcoma NOS**
	skin C460 soft tissue C461
	palate C462 lymph nodes C463
	gastrointestinal sites C464
	lung: unsp C4650 right C4651 left C4652
	other sites C467
B1089	**KSHVI: Kaposi's sarcoma associated herpes virus infection**
M963	**Kyphosis postlaminectomy**
M962	**Kyphosis postradiation**
-	**Labyrinthine hydrops - SEE Vertigo Meniere's**
E739	**Lactose intolerance NOS**
	congenital lactase deficiency E730
	secondary lactase deficiency E731
	other E738
-	**Lacunar syndromes**
	pure motor G465
	pure sensory G466
	other G467
G7080	**Lambert-Eaton syndrome NOS**
	in neoplastic disease G731 code neoplasm first
	in other disease G7081 code underlying disease first
J040	**Laryngitis acute**
	acute obstructive J050
J042	**Laryngotracheitis acute**
I447	**LBBB: left bundle branch block NOS**
	SEE Heart block for more
I4460	**LBBH: left bundle branch hemiblock NOS**
	SEE Heart block for more
M545	**LBP: low back pain**
R740	**LDH: lactic acid dehydrogenase elevated blood level**
L02415	**Leg abscess cutaneous right**
	left L02416
Z899	**Leg amputation status NOS**
	above knee: NOS Z89619 right Z89611 left Z89612
	at ankle: NOS Z89449 right Z89441 left Z89442
	at hip: NOS Z89629 right Z89621 left Z89622
	below knee: NOS Z89519 right Z89511 left Z89512
I724	**Leg artery aneurysm**
L02435	**Leg carbuncle right, code organism if known**
	left L02436
G5770	**Leg causalgia unsp**
	right G5771 left G5772
-	**Leg compartment syndrome**
	nontraumatic: right M79A21 left M79A22 unsp M79A29
	traumatic: right T79A21- left T79A22- unsp T79A29-
	For traumatic codes, 7th character indicates encounter
	A - initial encounter D - subsequent encounter S - sequela
	Includes all sites from hip to toes

R252	**Leg cramps NOS**
	sleep related G4762
	charley-horse M62831
	carpo-pedal spasm R290
Z86718	**Leg deep vein thrombosis personal history of**
R600	**Leg edema NOS**
I743	**Leg embolism arterial**
-	**Leg embolism/thrombosis venous deep ACUTE**
	unsp: right I82401 left I82402 bilat I82403 unsp I82409
	femoral: right I82411 left I82412 bilat I82413 unsp I82419
	iliac: right I82421 left I82422 bilat I82423 unsp I82429
	popliteal: right I82431 left I82432 bilat I82433 unsp I82439
	tibial: right I82441 left I82442 bilat I82443 unsp I82449
-	**Leg embolism/thrombosis venous deep CHRONIC**
	unsp: right I82501 left I82502 bilat I82503 unsp I82509
	femoral: right I82511 left I82512 bilat I82513 unsp I82519
	iliac: right I82521 left I82522 bilat I82523 unsp I82529
	popliteal: right I82531 left I82532 bilat I82533 unsp I82539
	tibial: right I82541 left I82542 bilat I82543 unsp I82549
-	**Leg fracture pathological NOS / (in neoplastic disease below)**
	femur unsp M84453- right M84451- left M84452-
	tibia right M84461- left M84462-
	fibula right M84463- left M84464-
	lowerleg unsp M84469-
	7th character indicates encounter/status
	A - initial S - sequela
	D - subsequent routine healing
	G - subsequent delayed healing
	K - subsequent nonunion P - subsequent malunion
	Change 4th character to 5 for 'in neoplastic disease'
L02425	**Leg furuncle/boil right**
	left L02426
R2240	**Leg lump/mass/swelling skin NOS**
	right R2241 left R2242 bilat R2243
G8310	**Leg monoplegia NOS**
	dominant side: right G8311 left G8312
	nondominant: right G8313 left G8314
-	**Leg osteonecrosis 4th character below**
	pelvis: M87-50
	femur: unsp M87-59 right M87-51 left M87-52
	tibia: unsp M87-63 right M87-61 left M87-62
	fibula: unsp M87-66 right M87-64 left M87-65
	ankle: unsp M87-73 right M87-71 left M87-72
	foot: unsp M87-76 right M87-74 left M87-75
	toes: unsp M87-79 right M87-77 left M87-78
	4th character
	idiopathic aseptic = 0 d/t drugs = 1 d/t trauma = 2
	other secondary = 3 other = 8

-	**Leg osteoporosis age related w/current pathological fracture**
	femur: unsp M80059- right M80051- left M80052-
	lower leg: unsp M80069- right M80061- left M80062-
	ankle / foot: unsp M80079- right M80071- left M80072-
	7th character indicates encounter/status
	A - initial S - sequela
	D - subsequent routine healing
	G - subsequent delayed healing
	K - subsequent nonunion P - subsequent malunion
I743	**Leg peripheral disease occlusive**
-	**Leg varicose veins calf**
	w/ulcer: unspec I83001 right I83012 left I83022
	w/inflammation: unspec I8310 right I8311 left I8312
	inflammation only code apply to any part of leg
	w/inflammation & ulcer: unspec I83202 right I83212 left I83222
	code to identify severity of ulcer below
	skin breakdown: right L97211 left L97221 unsp L97201
	fat exposed: right L97212 left L97222 unsp L97202
	muscle necrosis: right L97213 left L97223 unsp L97203
	bone necrosis: right L97214 left L97224 unsp L97204
	unspecified: right L97219 left L97229 unsp L97209
I8390	**Leg varicose veins NOS**
	right I8391 left I8392 bilat I8393
A481	**Legionnaires' disease**
	nonpneumonic Legionnaire's disease A482
-	**Lemoyez' syndrome SEE vertigo peripheral NOS**
I673	**Leukoecephalopathy progressive vascular**
I456	**LGL: Lown-Ganong-Levine syndrome**
R87612	**LGSIL: low grade squamous intraepithelial lesion from cervix pap smear**
	from vaginal pap smear R87622
I501	**LHF: left heart failure NOS**
M3211	**Libman-Sacks disease**
B852	**Lice NOS**
	body B851 head B850
	pubic B853
	mixed infection B854
L439	**Lichen planus unsp**
	hypertrophic L430 bullous L431
	lichenoid drug rection L432
	subacute / tropicus L433
	other L438
R42	**Lightheaded**
K4090	**LIH: left inguinal hernia NOS -- SEE INGUINAL HERNIA FOR MORE**
K750	**Liver abscess NOS**

K7460	**Liver cirrhosis NOS**
	alcoholic: NOS K7030 w/ascites K7031
	other/ cryptogenic/ portal/ postnecrotic K7469
	pigmentary E83110
	w/ toxic liver disease K717
	RELATED esophageal varices I8510 w/bleeding I8511
K761	**Liver congestion chronic passive**
K709	**Liver disease alcoholic NOS**
-	**Liver failure**
	acute/ subacute: NOS K7200 w/coma K7201
	chronic: NOS K7210 w/coma K7211
	unsp: NOS K7290 w/coma K7291
K7040	**Liver failure alcoholic NOS**
	w/coma K7041
K760	**Liver fatty NEC**
	alcoholic K700
K740	**Liver fibrosis**
	w/ sclerosis K742
K702	**Liver fibrosis & sclerosis alcoholic**
K763	**Liver infarction**
K739	**Liver inflammation NOS**
	supperative K750
K762	**Liver necrosis central hemorrhagic**
	if with hepatic failure, included in Liver failure code
-	**Liver neoplasms**
	MALIGNANT primary
	liver cell carcinoma / hepatoma C220
	intrahepatic bile duct carcinoma C221
	hepatoblastoma C222
	angiosarcoma C223 other sarcoma C224
	other carcinoma C227
	primary unsp type C228
	not specified primary or secondary / NOS C229
	Secondary C787 Benign D134
	Mets to bone C7951 mets to unsp lymph nodes C779
K741	**Liver sclerosis**
	w/ fibrosis K742
R55	**LOC: loss of consciousness no trauma NOS (blackout)**
G835	**Locked-in state**
I4581	**Long QT syndrome**
-	**Long term use (current) medications - includes aftercare NEC**
	methadone for pain Z79891
	antibiotics Z792 aspirin Z7982
	anticoagulants Z7901 systemic steroids Z7951
	antiplatelet / antithrombotic Z7902
	nonsteroidal antiinflammatories Z791

-	**Lordosis acquired**
	unsp: unsp M4050 thoracolumbar M4055
	unsp: lumbar M4056 lumbosacral M4057
	postural: unsp M4040 thoracolumbar M4055
	postural: lumbar M4046 lumbosacral M4047
	postop M964
M545	**Lumbago unsp**
	w/sciatica: unsp M5440 right M5441 left M5442
-	**Lumbar neuritis or radiculitis SEE Radiculopathy**
-	**Lumbar puncture complication**
	fluid leak G970 headache G971
	hemorrhage/hematoma G9751
J852	**Lung abscess NOS**
	w/pneumonia J851
J850	**Lung gangrene & necrosis**
-	**Lung neoplasm (and bronchus)**
	MALIGNANT primary
	bronchus: unsp C3400 right C3401 left C3402
	upper lobe bronchus or lung: unsp C3410 right C3411 left C3412
	lower lobe bronchus or lung: unsp C3430 right C3431 left C3432
	middle lobe C342
	overlapping sites bronchus & lung: unsp C3480 right C3481 left C3482
	unspecified part bronchus or lung: unsp C3490 right C3491 left C3492
	Secondary: unsp lung C7800 right C7801 left C7802
	Benign: unsp D1430 right D1431 left D1432
	Mets to bone C7951 mets to unsp lymph nodes C779
L930	**Lupus erythematosus non systemic NOS**
	subacute cutaneous L931
	other L932
M329	**Lupus erythematosus systemic NOS**
	Drug induced M320 w/lung involvement M3213
	w/endocarditis M3211 w/pericarditis M3212
	w/tubulo-interstitial disease M3215
	w/glomerular disease M3214
	w/other organ or system involvement M3219
	other forms of SLE M328
-	**LUTS: lower urinary tract symptoms -Code first any cause eg BPH**
	Code also any associated overactive bladder N3281
	bladder incomplete emptying R3914
	nocturia physical R351 psychogenic F458
	straining on urination R3916
	urinary frequency R350
	urinary hesitancy R3911
	urinary incontinence NOS R32 see urinary incontinence for more
	urinary obstruction N139
	urinary retention R339
	urinary urgency N3941 weak urinary stream R3912

A6920	**Lyme disease unsp**
	meningitis A6921 other neurologic disorder A6922
	arthritis A6923 other A6929
-	**Lymph node neoplasms SECONDARY**
	AS METS FROM OTHER NEOPLASMS
	head / face / neck C770
	intrathoracic C771
	intra-abdominal C772
	axilla / arm C773
	inguinal / leg C774
	intrapelvic C775
	multiple regions C778
	unsp / NOS C779
I889	**Lymphadenitis NOS**
	acute unsp L049 chronic except mesentery I881
	mesenteric unsp I880
	d/t brugia (wuchereria) malayi B741
	d/t wuchereria bancroftia B740
	acute: face/neck L040 trunk L041
	acute: arm / axilla L042 leg L043
R591	**Lymphadenopathy NOS**
	same code for generalized enlarged lymph nodes
	localized enlarged nodes R590
	enlarged nodes unsp R599
I891	**Lymphangitis chronic / NOS**
I890	**Lymphedema acquired/praecox/secondary NOS**
	postmastectomy I972
I898	**Lymphocele any site**
	also chylous ascites, chylous cyst, lymph node rupture
-	**Lymphoma non-Hodgkin / NOS / malignant**
	unsp site C8590 head/face/neck C8591 intrathoracic C8592
	intra-abdominal C8593 axilla / arm C8594 inguinal / leg C8595
	intrapelvic C8596 spleen C8597 multiple C8598 extranodal C8599
A319	**MAC/MTB: mycobacterium avium complex infection NOS / atypical**
	pulmonary A310
-	**Machine dependence**
	respirator Z9911 aspirator Z990
	cardiac pacemaker Z950
	supplemental oxygen Z9981
	wheel chair Z993
	heart assist device Z95811
	AICD Z95810
	renal dialysis Z992
H3530	**Macular degeneration senile NOS**
	exudative H3532 non-exudative H3531
E8340	**Magnesium metabolism disorder NOS**
	hypermagnesemia E8341
	hypomagnesemia E8342
	other E8349

K909	**Malabsorption syndrome NOS**
	following GI surgery K912
	of disaccharides E7439
E46	**Malnutrition NOS**
	kwashiorkor E40 marasmic kwashiorkor E42
	nutritional marasmus E41
	protein-calorie severe NOS E43 moderate E440 mild E441
	retarded development d/t E45
E710	**Maple syrup urine disease**
C7952	**Marrow neoplasm SECONDARY / Mets to marrow**
	to bone C7951
-	**Mastoiditis acute**
	NOS: right H70001 left H70002
	bilat H70003 unsp H70009
	w/abscess: right H70011 left H70012
	bilat H70013 unsp H70019
	w/other complication: right H70091 left H70092
	bilat H70093 unsp H70099
-	**Mastoiditis chronic NOS and UNSP and in infectious disease**
	chronic: unsp H7010 bilat H7013
	chronic: right H7011 left H7012
	unsp: unsp H7090 bilat H7093
	unsp: right H7091 left H7092
	in infectious / parasitic disease classified elsewhere --
	unsp H7500 bilat H7503 right H7501 left H7502
N6019	**Mastopathy diffuse cystic**
	right N6011 left N6012
I671	**MCA: middle cerebral aneurysm**
G3184	**MCI: mild cognitive impairment, so stated**
M303	**MCLS: mucocutaneous lymph node syndrome**
H3530	**MD: macular degeneration NOS (age related)**
	exudative H3532 non-exudative H3531
G710	**MD: muscular dystrophy except myotonic or CMT type**
	mytonic G7111
F339	**MDD: major depressive disorder recurrent episode NOS**
	mild F330 moderate F331
	severe F332 severe w/psychotic behavior F333
	in remission NOS F3340
	full remission F3342 partial remission F3341
	recurrent brief episodes F338
F329	**MDD: major depressive disorder single episode NOS**
	mild F320 moderate F321
	severe NOS F322 severe w/psychotic behavior F323
	partial or unspecified remission F324
	in full remission F325
D469	**MDS: myelodysplastic syndrome NOS**
N342	**Meatitis urethral**
-	**Medication monitoring SEE Drug level monitoring**

-	**Medications long term use (current)** - includes aftercare
	SEE Drug Long term use
-	**Mediport infection**
	systemic infection T80211-
	local infection T80212-
	other spec T80218-
	unsp T80219-
	7th character indicates encounter
	A - initial encounter D - subsequent encounter S - sequela
	includes Hickman, PIC, portacath, triple lumen etc
K593	**Megacolon NEC**
	in Chaga's disease B5732
	in Clostridiium difficile A047
	in Hirschsprung's disease Q431
N2882	**Megaloureter**
-	**Melanoma malignant**
	lip C430 scalp & neck C434
	eyelid: unsp C4310 right C4311 left C4312
	ear: unsp C4320 right C4321 left C4322
	nose C4331 face NOS C4330 other parts of face C4339
	trunk: anal skin C4351 breast C4352 other C4359
	arm/shoulder: unsp C4360 right C4361 left C4362
	leg/hip: unsp C4370 right C4371 left C4372
	overlapping sites C438
	unsp / NOS C439
	Mets to bone C7951 mets to unsp lymph nodes C779
E8841	**MELAS: mitochondrial encephalopathy, lactic acidosis and stroke like episodes**
K921	**Melena**
R413	**Memory loss NOS**
Z1581	**MEN: multiple endocrine neoplasia genetic susceptibility**
E3120	**MEN: multiple endocrine neoplasia NOS**
	type I E3121 type IIA E3122 type IIB E3123
Z8341	**MEN: multiple endocrine neoplasia syndrome family history of**
-	**Meninges neoplasm malignant primary**
	cerebral meninges C700 secondary C7932 benign D320
	spinal meninges C701 secondary C7949 benign D321
	unspecified C709 secondary C7949 benign D329
G000	**Meningitis bacterial hemophilus influenzae**
G01	**Meningitis bacterial in other disease NEC**
	RELATED UNDERLYING
	leptospirosis A2781 listeriosis A3211
	meningococcal A390 neurosyphilis A5213
	tuberculosis A170 gonococcal A5481

G009	**Meningitis bacterial NOS**
	nonpyogenic NOS G030
	chronic NOS G031
	benign recurrent NOS G032
	d/t other specified causes G038
	in other bacterial disease G01
	in other infectius disease G02
	meningitis unsp G039
G008	**Meningitis bacterial other**
G001	**Meningitis bacterial pneumococcal**
G003	**Meningitis bacterial staphylococcal**
G002	**Meningitis bacterial streptococcal**
B375	**Meningitis candidal**
G02	**Meningitis nonbacterial in other infectious/parasitic disease**
	RELATED UNDERLYING candidal B375
	cryptococcal B451 herpes simplex B003
	measles complicated by meningitis B051
	mumps meningitis B261 varicella meningitis B010
	rubella meningitis B0602 zoster meningitis B021
	coccidioidomycosis B384
A879	**Meningitis viral NOS**
	enteroviral A870 adenoviral A871
	lymphocytic choriomeningitis A872
	other A878
-	**Meningococcal infections**
	unspecified A399 meningitis A390
	adrenal syndrome A391 meningoccemia unsp A394
	meningococcemia acute A392 meningococcemia chronic A393
	carditis unsp A3950 endocarditis A3951
	myocarditis A3952 pericarditis A3953
	encephalitis A3981 retrobulbar neuritis A3982
	arthritis A3983 postmeningococcal arthritis A3984
	conjunctivitis A3989
E28319	**Menopause premature asymptomatic**
	symptomatic E28310
E8842	**MERRF: myoclonic epilepsy associated with ragged red fibers syndrome**
I880	**Mesenteric lymphadenitis acute/chronic/subacute**
C459	**Mesothelioma unsp**
	of pleura C450
	of peritoneum C451
	includes mesentery, mesocolon, omentum
	of pericardium C452
	other sites C457
R948	**Metabolism basal abnormal**
I213	**MI: myocardial infarction NOS (any current episode)**
I252	**MI: old myocardial infarction (over 1 year)**

-	**Micturition difficulty**
	hesitancy R3911
	weak stream R3912
	split stream R3913
	incomplete bladder emptying R3914
	urgency R3915
	straining R3916
	other R3919
C717	**Midbrain neoplasm malignant primary**
	Secondary C7931 Benign D331
G43D0	**Migraine abdominal NOS**
	intractable G43D1
G43709	**Migraine chronic w/o aura NOS**
	w/status migrainosus G43701
	intractable NOS G43719
	intractable w/status migrainosus G43711
G43009	**Migraine common NOS**
	w/status migrainosus G43001
	intractable NOS G43019
	intractable w/status migrainosus G43011
G43829	**Migraine menstrual NOS**
	w/status migrainosus G43821
	intractable NOS G43839
	intractable w/status migrainosus G43831
G43909	**Migraine NOS**
	w/status migrainosus G43901
	intractable NOS G43919
	intractable w/status migrainosus G43911
G43109	**Migraine w/aura, classical NOS**
	w/status migrainosus G43101
	intractable NOS G43119
	intractable w/status migrainosus G43111
I349	**Mitral valve disorder nonrheumatic unsp**
	insufficiency I340 prolapse I341
	stenosis I342 other I348
B2790	**MONO: mononucleosis infectious NOS**
	SEE mononucleosis for more
B2790	**Mononucleosis infectious NOS**
	w/polyneuropathy B2791
	w/meningitis B2792
	w/complication other B2799
	Change 4th character if type of virus is specified:
	gammaherpesviral = 0
	cytomegaloviral = 1
	other specified = 8
	RELATED hepatitis K77
	RELATED encephalitis G053

G8330	**Monoplegia NOS**
	dominant side: right G8331 left G8332
	nondominant: right G8333 left G8334
	SEE ARM or LEG if specified
I675	**Moyamoya disease**
A812	**MPL: multifocal progressive leukoencephalopathy**
E761	**MPS: mucopolysaccharidosis type II**
	NOS E763 type I Hurler's E7601
	type I Hurler-Scheie E7602
	type I Scheie's E7603
	Morquio A E76210 Morquio B E76211
	Morquio unsp E76219
	Sanfilippo E7622
	other spec E7629
I52	**MPSC: mucopolysaccharidosis cardiopathy**
	Code first mucopolysaccharidosis, "MPS"
F79	**MR: mental retardation NOS SEE ID for more**
A4902	**MRSA: methicillin resistant staph aureus infection (not sepsis)**
	MRSA as cause of other disease B9562
A4102	**MRSAS: methicillin resistant staph aureus septicemia / sepsis**
G35	**MS: multiple sclerosis**
B9561	**MSSA: methicillin susceptible staph aureus as cause of disease**
A4101	**MSSAS: methicillin susceptible staph aureus septicemia**
	MRSSAS methicillin resistant staph aureus sepsis A4102
K1230	**Mucositis oral unsp**
	ulcerative d/t antineoplastic therapy K1231
	ulcerative d/t other drugs K1232
	ulcerative d/t radiation K1233
	other K1239
C9000	**Multiple myeloma NOS**
	in remission C9001
	in relapse C9002
G35	**Multiple sclerosis**
B269	**Mumps NOS**
	orchitis B260 meningitis B261
	encephalitis B262 pancreatitis B263
	hepatitis B2681 myocarditis B2682
	nephritis B2683 polyneuropathy B2684
	arthritis B2685 other complications B2689
G710	**Muscular dystrophy**
	mytonic G7111
J675	**Mushroom worker's lung**
I349	**MVD: mitral valve disease NOS**
	rheumatic I059
I341	**MVP: mitral valve prolapse NOS**
I340	**MVR: mitral valve regurgitation NOS**
G7000	**Myasthenia gravis NOS**
	w/acute exacerbation G7001

-	**Mycosis fungoides**
	unsp site C8400 head/face/neck C8401 intrathoracic C8402
	intra-abdominal C8403 axilla / arm C8404 inguinal / leg C8405
	intrapelvic C8406 spleen C8407 multiple C8408 extranodal C8409
B0112	**Myelitis in chickenpox**
B0224	**Myelitis in herpes zoster**
G0491	**Myelitis NOS**
	transverse G373 toxic G92
	postinfectious other G054
	herpes: zoster B0224 simplex B0082
	postimmunization G0402
	post chickenpox B0112
I515	**Myocardial degeneration**
I213	**Myocardial infarction acute NOS**
	acute subendocardial / non-Q wave NOS I214
I214	**Myocardial infarction non-ST elevated (non STEMI)**
I252	**Myocardial infarction old**
I510	**Myocardial infarction sequelae cardiac septal defect old**
	as current complication following MI:
	atrial septal defect I231
	ventricular septal defect I232
I213	**Myocardial infarction ST elevated NOS (STEMI)**
	left main coronary artery I2101
	left anterior descending coronary artery I2102
	other coronary artery of anterior wall I2109
	right coronary artery I2111
	other coronary artery of inferior wall I2119
	left circumflex coronary artery I2121
	other sites I2129
-	**Myocardial infarction SUBSEQUENT within 4 weeks of previous**
	STEMI anterior wall I220
	STEMI inferior wall I221
	NSTEMI NOS I222
	STEMI other sites I228
	STEMI NOS I229
I240	**Myocardial ischemia acute w/MI**
I401	**Myocarditis acute/subacute giant cell / Fiedler's/ idiopathic/ isolated**
	acute NOS I409
	NOS / chronic interstitial I514
	septic I400 other I408
	rheumatic: NOS I090 acute I012
	gonococcal A5483
G253	**Myoclonus**
G709	**Myoneural disorder NOS**

G729	**Myopathy NOS**
	inflammatory NOS G7249
	critical illness G7281
	alcoholic G721 drug induced G720
	d/t other toxic agent G722 code agent first
	hereditary NOS G719
E039	**Myxedema NOS**
	coma E035
R112	**N&V: nausea and vomiting together**
K760	**NAFLD: nonalcoholic fatty liver disease**
-	**Nail disorders**
	ingrowing L600 onycholysis L601
	onychogryphosis L602 dystrophy L603
	Beau's lines L604 yellow nail syndrome L605
	other L608 unspecified L609
E8849	**NARP: neuropathy, ataxia and retinitis pigmentosa syndrome**
K7581	**NASH: nonalcoholic steatohepatitis**
R110	**Nausea NOS**
	with vomiting R11.2
G4452	**NDPH: new daily persistent headache**
K550	**NEC: necrotizing enterocolitis**
-	**Neoplasm secondary, mets from other**
	abdominal / hepatic / splenic C772 axillary C773
	cervical / neck C770 esophageal, diaphragmatic C771
	groin / popliteal C774 intrapelvic C775
	multiple sites C778 unspecified C779
N009	**Nephritic syndrome acute unsp**
	w/minor glomerular abnormality N000
	w/focal & segmental glomerular lesions N001
	w/diffuse membranous glomerulonephritis N002
	w/diffuse mesangial proliferative glomerulonephritis N003
	w/diffuse endocapillary proliferative glomerulonephritis N004
	w/diffuse mesangiocapillary glomerulonephritis N005
	w/dense deposit disease N006
	w/diffuse crescentic glomerulonephritis N007
	w/other morphologic changes N008
	CHANGE third character to 1 for 'Rapidly Progressive' N. syndrome
N039	**Nephritic syndrome chronic unsp**
	w/minor glomerular abnormality N030
	w/focal & segmental glomerular lesions N031
	w/diffuse membranous glomerulonephritis N032
	w/diffuse mesangial proliferative glomerulonephritis N033
	w/diffuse endocapillary proliferative glomerulonephritis N034
	w/diffuse mesangiocapillary glomerulonephritis N035
	w/dense deposit disease N036
	w/diffuse crescentic glomerulonephritis N037
	w/other morphologic changes N038
	CHANGE third character to 5 for 'Unspecified' N. syndrome

N059	**Nephritis NOS**
	w/renal cortical necrosis N171
	salt-losing N2889
	chronic NOS N039 acute NOS N009
N200	**Nephrolithiasis NOS**
	w/ureter calculus N202
N289	**Nephropathy NOS**
N144	**Nephropathy Toxic NEC**
	analgesic N140
	d/t other drug N141
	d/t unspec drug N142
	heavy metal N143
N2883	**Nephroptosis**
Z436	**Nephrostomy care**
N08	**Nephrotic syndrome IN:**
	amyloidosis/ diabetes mellitus/ malaria
	polyarteritis/ systemic lupus
N049	**Nephrotic syndrome unsp**
	w/minor glomerular abnormality N040
	w/focal & segmental glomerular lesions N041
	w/diffuse membranous glomerulonephritis N042
	w/diffuse mesangial proliferative glomerulonephritis N043
	w/diffuse endocapillary proliferative glomerulonephritis N044
	w/diffuse mesangiocapillary glomerulonephritis N045
	w/dense deposit disease N046
	w/diffuse crescentic glomerulonephritis N047
	w/other morphologic changes N048
T148	**Nerve injury peripheral NOS**
	abdomen / lower back / pelvis S346xx-
	neck S144xx-
	7th character indicates encounter
	A - initial encounter D - subsequent encounter S - sequela
G609	**Neuropathy hereditary/idiopathic NOS**
	idiopathic progressive G603
	hereditary motor & senory G600
Q8500	**NF: neurofibromatosis unspecified**
	NF1 type I Q8501 NF2 type II 8502
	other NF Q8509 Schwannomatosis Q8503
N341	**NGU: non-gonococcal urethritis NOS**
E119	**NIDDM: non-insulin dependent diabetes mellitus type 2 NOS**
	SEE Diabetes type 2 for more
E75249	**Niemann-Pick disease NOS**
	type A E75240 type B E75241
	type C E75242 type D E75243
	other E75248
E1101	**NKHHC: nonketotic hyperglycemic-hyperosmolar coma in Type 2 diabetes**
R351	**Nocturia**

J339	**Nose polyp unsp**
	nasal cavity / choanal J330
	polypoid degeneration J331
	of sinus J338
G912	**NPH: normal pressure hydrocephalus**
	G910 secondary
B9629	**NSTEC: non-shiga toxin producing e coli as cause of disease**
I214	**NSTEMI: non-ST elevation myocardial infaction NOS**
	SEE myocardial infarction for more
-	**Nucleus palposus herniated**
	cervical NOS M5030
	lumbar M5136
	thoracic M5134
M1990	**OA: osteoarthritis unsp site NOS - SEE site for specific**
	primary NOS M1991
	post-traumatic NOS M1992
	secondary NOS M1993
E669	**Obese NOS also code BMI if known**
	d/t excess calories: NOS E6609 morbid E6601
	drug induced E661
	morbid w/alveolar hypoventilation E662
	overweight NOS E663
	other obesity E668
F09	**OBS: organic brain syndrome NOS**
F42	**OCD: obsessive compulsive disorder**
E662	**OHS: obesity hypoventilation syndrome (Pickwickian)**
H6690	**OM: otitis media NOS include acute / chronic NOS**
	right H6691 left H6692 bilateral H6693
L0882	**Omphalitis not of newborn**
N7092	**Oophoritis unsp**
	acute N7002
	chronic N7012
G238	**OPCA: olivopontocerebellar atrophy**
-	**Orthopedic aftercare**
	Z471 following joint replacement surgery
	Z472 for removal of internal fixation device
	Z4733 following explantation of knee joint prosthesis
	Z4732 following explantation of hip joint prosthesis
	Z4731 following explantation of shoulder joint prosthesis
	Z4782 following scoliosis surgery
	Z4781 following surgical amputation
	Use additional code to identify limb amputated (Z89.-)
	Z4789 other orthopedic aftercare
Z4689	**Orthopedic brace fitting & adjustment**
G4733	**OSA: obstructive sleep apnea (adult or child)**

M839	**Osteomalacia adult unsp**
	puerperal M830 senile M831
	d/t malabsorption M832
	d/t malnutrition M833
	aluminum bone disease M834
	other drug induced M835
	other specified M838
M810	**Osteoporosis NOS (no current fracture)**
	age-related/ postmenopausal/ senile M810
	drug induced / disuse / postpro / post-trauma M818
	localized M816
	Personal history of (healed) osteoporosis fracture Z87310
	with current fracture SEE site
Z5189	**OT: occupational therapy**
-	**Otitis externa**
	candidal B3784
	diffuse: right H60311 left H60312 bilateral H60313 unsp H60319
	Using diffuse codes as guide:
	If specified other infective change 5th character to '9'
	If specified swimmers ear change 5th character to '3'
	If specified hemorrhagic change 5th character to '2'
	acute noninfective NOS:
	right H60501 left H60502 bilateral H60503 unspecified H60519
-	**Otitis media acute & subacute allergic**
	NOS: unsp H65119 right H65111 left H65112 bilat H65113
	recurrent: unsp H65117 right H65114 left H65115 bilat H65116
-	**Otitis media acute & subacute mucoid / nonsuppurative NOS**
	NOS: unsp H65199 right H65191 left H65192 bilat H65193
	recurrent: unsp H65197 right H65194 left H65195 bilat H65196
-	**Otitis media acute serous**
	NOS: unsp H6500 right H6501 left H6502 bilat H6503
	recurrent: unsp H6507 right H6504 left H6505 bilat H6506
-	**Otitis media CHRONIC**
	serous: unsp H6520 right H6521 left H6522 bilat H6523
	mucoid: unsp H6530 right H6531 left H6532 bilat H6533
	allergic: unsp H65419 right H65411 left H65412 bilat H65413
-	**Otitis media UNSP as acute or chronic**
	unsp H6690 right H6691 left H6692 bilat H6693
N8331	**Ovary atrophy acquired**
N8320	**Ovary cysts unspecified**
	follicular N830
	corpus luteum N831
	other N8329

-	**Ovary neoplasm**
	Malignant primary: unsp C569 right C561 left C562
	Secondary: unsp C7960 right C7961 left C7962
	Benign: unsp D279 right D270 left D271
	Mets to bone C7951 mets to unsp lymph nodes C779
	Mets to intraabdominal lymph node C772
	Mets to intrapelvic lymph node C775
E282	**Ovary polycystic**
N8351	**Ovary torsion**
-	**Overweight - SEE obese**
I491	**PAC: premature atrial contraction**
-	**Pacemaker complication**
	Embolism T82817-
	Pain T82847-
	Infection and inflammatory reaction T827xx-
	Use additional code to identify infection
	hemorrhage T82837-
	7th character indicates encounter
	A - initial encounter D - subsequent encounter S - sequela
Z45018	**Pacemaker fitting & adjustment**
	check / test / replace pacemaker battery Z45010
Z95.0	**Pacemaker status**
I498	**Pacemaker wandering**
I480	**PAF: paroxysmal atrial fibrillation**
I4892	**PAF: paroxysmal atrial flutter**
R52	**Pain NOS**
	post-thoracotomy: acute G8912 chronic G8922
	other postop: acute G8918 chronic G8928
	d/t trauma: acute G8911 chronic G8921
	neoplasm related G893 chronic pain syndrome G894
	SEE also backache, headache, migraine, abdominal
R309	**Pain on urination NOS**
	dysuria R300
G890	**Pain syndrome central**
G894	**Pain syndrome chronic**
-	**Pain syndrome complex regional**
	CRPS I
	arm: right G90511 left G90512 bilat G90513 NOS G90519
	leg: right G90521 left G90522 bilat G90523 NOS G90529
	other site G9059 unsp G9050
	CRPS II
	leg: right G5771 left G5772 NOS G5770
	arm: right G5641 left G5642 NOS G5640

C059	**Palate neoplasm malignant primary unsp**
	hard palate C050 uvula C052
	soft palate C051 overlapping sites C058
	SECONDARY all C7989 BENIGN all D1039
	Mets to bone C7951
	Mets to axilla / arm lymph node C773
	mets to esophageal nodes C771
Z515	**Palliative care**
M300	**PAN: polyarteritis nodosa NOS**
	with lung involvement M301 juvenile M302
K859	**Pancreas abscess/(acute necrosis) SEE Pancreatitis for more**
K862	**Pancreas cyst**
	pseudocyst K863
K868	**Pancreas disorders**
	atrophy cirrhosis fibrosis insufficiency necrosis
	Same code for all
C259	**Pancreas neoplasm malignant primary NOS**
	overlapping sites C258
	head C250 body C251
	tail C252 pancreatic duct C253
	endocrine / islets of Langerhans C254
	other parts C257
	Secondary C7889
	Benign: endocrine D137 all other D136
	Mets to bone C7951 mets to unsp lymph nodes C779
	mets to abdominal lymph nodes C772
K863	**Pancreas pseudocyst**
	cyst K862
K859	**Pancreatitis acute NOS**
	incl hemorrhagic/necrotic/ NOS/ subacute/ suppurative
	idiopathic acute K850 biliary acute K851
	alcohol induced acute K852
	drug induced acute K853
	other acute K858
K861	**Pancreatitis chronic NOS**
	incl infectious/ painless/ recurrent/ relapsing
	alcohol induced chronic K860
K868	**Pancreatolithiasis**
D61818	**Pancytopenia other**
	d/t antineoplastic chemotherapy D61810
	d/t other drug D61811
J189	**PAP: primary atypical pneumonia**
R295	**Paralysis transient**
G839	**Paralytic syndrome unsp**
G8220	**Paraplegia NOS**
	complete G8221 incomplete G8222
G20	**Parkinson's disease idiopathic/NOS/primary**
	dementia w/Parkinsonism G3183

G219	**Parkinsonism secondary unsp**
	malignant neuroleptic syndrome G210
	neuroleptic induced G2111 other drug induced G2119
	d/t other external agents G212 vascular G214
	postencephalitic G213 other secondary G218
C07	**Parotid gland neoplasm malignant primary**
	secondary C7989 benign D110
	Mets to bone C7951 mets to unsp lymph nodes C779
	mets to esophageal nodes C771
I471	**PAT: paroxysmal atrial tachycardia**
-	**Patella disorders**
	recurrent dislocate: unsp M2200 right M2201 left M2202
	recurrent sublux: unsp M2210 right M2211 left M2212
	other derangements: unsp M223x9 right M223x1 left M223x2
	chondromalacia: unsp M2240 right M2241 left M2242
	other disorder: unsp M228x9 right M228x1 left M228x2
	unsp disorder: unsp M2290 right M2291 left M2292
-	**Patient education**
	diabetes/ diet/ obesity Z713
	exercise / injury prevention Z7189
	insulin pump Z4681
	medications / treatment plan Z7189
	tobacco abuse counseling Z716
R3989	**PBS: painful bladder syndrome**
E282	**PCOS: polycystic ovary syndrome**
B59	**PCP: pneumonia/pneumocytosis d/t pneumocystis carinii/jiroveci**
D45	**PCV: polycythemia vera**
R600	**Pedal edema**
-	**PEDICULOSIS - SEE lice**
N733	**Pelvis abscess female acute**
	chronic N734 NOS N735
-	**Pelvis abscess MALE SEE Peritonitis**
N736	**Pelvis adhesions female postinfective**
	postop N994 (male / female)
-	**Pelvis bone cyst**
	solitary cyst: unsp M85459 right M85451 left M85452
	aneurysmal cyst: change 4th character to 5
	other cyst: change 4th character to 6
N9489	**Pelvis congestion syndrome**
N803	**Pelvis endometriosis (pelvic peritoneum) female**
M84454-	**Pelvis fracture pathological NOS / in neoplastic disease**
	Change 4th character to 5 for 'in neoplastic disease'
	7th character indicates encounter/status
	A - initial S - sequela
	D - subsequent routine healing
	G - subsequent delayed healing
	K - subsequent nonunion P - subsequent malunion
N8182	**Pelvis fundus incompetence/weakening**

N739	**Pelvis inflammatory disease NOS (female)**
	gonococcal A5424
	chlamydial A5611
N739	**Pelvis inflammatory disease NOS female**
	chronic N731
	acute N730
	in other disease N74 See a few below
	RELATED UNDERLYING diseases - code first
	tuberculous A1817
	chlamydia trachomatis A5611
	syphilitic (secondary) A5276
	gonococcal pelvic inflammatory disease A5424
	herpes simplex pelvic inflammatory disease A6009
	trichomoniasis A5909
N8184	**Pelvis muscle wasting female**
R102	**Pelvis pain NOS**
R1900	**Pelvis swelling, mass, lump NOS**
	Generalized R1907 Other R1909
I862	**Pelvis varices**
L109	**Pemphigus NOS**
	vulgaris L100 vegetans L101
	foliaceous L102 Brazilian L103
	erythematosus L104 drug induced L105
	paraneoplastic L1081 other L1089
K279	**Peptic ulcer NOS used with no site given or gastroduodenal**
	acute: w/hemorrhage K270 w/perforation K271
	acute: NOS K273 w/both hemorrhage/perforation K272
	chronic/unsp: w/hemorrhage K274 w/perforation K275
	chronic/unsp w/both hemorrhage/perforation K276
	chronic NOS K277
K610	**Perianal abscess / cellulitis**
I313	**Pericardial effusion noninflammatory**
	acute NOS I309
I319	**Pericarditis NOS**
	acute nonspecific idiopathic I300
	acute infective I301 acute unsp I309
	other acute I308
	chronic adhesive I310
	chronic constrictive I311
	in other disease I32
-	**Perichondritis ear external**
	right: NOS H61001 acute H61011 chronic H61021
	left: NOS H61002 acute H61012 chronic H61022
	bilat: NOS H61003 acute H61013 chronic H61023
	unsp: NOS H61009 acute H61019 chronic H61029
R102	**Perineal pain NOS**
N8181	**Perineocele**
L02215	**Perineum abscess cutaneous**
N340	**Perineum abscess deep w/urethral involvement**

L02225	**Perineum boil / furuncle**
L02235	**Perineum carbuncle**
B356	**Perineum infection fungal**
R579	**Peripheral circulation failure**
R600	**Peripheral edema pitting/dependent/NOS localized**
I872	**Peripheral insufficiency venous NOS**
I739	**Peripheral vascular disease NOS**
N736	**Peritoneal pelvic adhesions postinfective / NOS female**

    postop N994

- **Peritoneum & retroperitoneum neoplasm**
    MALIGNANT primary
    retroperitoneum C480
    specified parts of peritoneum C481
    peritoneum unsp / NOS C482
    overlapping sites of peritoneum & retroperitoneum C488
    SECONDARY both C786
    Retroperitoneum benign D200
    Peritoneum benign D201
    Mets to bone C7951   mets to unsp lymph nodes C779
    Mets to intraabdominal lymph node C772

K659	**Peritonitis NOS / acute NOS / bacterial NOS**

    chronic proliferative or d/t urine K658
    d/t bile K653   spontaneous bacterial K652
    generalized: acute K650 w/acute appendicitis K352
    gonococcal A5485
    female pelvic NOS N735
    SEE pelvis inflammatory disease for more

R1033	**Periumbilical pain**
N340	**Periurethral abscess**
R233	**Petechiae**
G547	**Phantom limb syndrome NOS**

    w/ pain G546

J029	**Pharyngitis acute NOS**

    chronic J312
    streptococcal J020
    w/ unsp flu NOS J111

G3101	**Pick's disease**

    RELATED dementia NOS F0280
    RELATED dementia w/behavioral disturbance F0281

E662	**Pickwickian syndrome**
-	**PID: prolapsed intervertebral disc w/myelopathy**

    thoracic M5104
    thoracolumbar M5105
    lumbar M5106

J82	**PIE: pulmonary infiltration w/eosinophilia**
-	**Pilonidal cyst and sinus**

    cyst NOS L0591   w/abscess L0501
    sinus/fistula NOS L0592   w/abscess L0502

-		**PIN: prostate intraepithelial neoplasia**
		type I or II or NOS (histologically confirmed) N423
		type III D075
B80	**Pinworm**	
		RELATED vaginitis / vulvitis N771
E236	**Pituitary abscess**	
E230	**Pituitary cachexia / insufficiency NOS**	
		postpro E893
		drug induced E231
E229	**Pituitary hyperfunction NOS**	
L42	**Pityriasis rosea**	
D552	**PK: (or PKA) pyruvate kinase deficiency anemia**	
E700	**PKU: phenylketonuria**	
G5760	**Plantar nerve lesion NOS**	
		right G5761 left G5762
B070	**Plantar warts**	
N943	**PMDD: premenstrual dysphoric / tension disorder**	
		see related migraines at PMS
A812	**PML: progressive multifocal leukoencephalopathy**	
M353	**PMR: polymyalgia rheumatica**	
		with giant cell arteritis M315
N943	**PMS: premenstrual syndrome (tension)**	
		RELATED Migraines
		not intractable: NOS G43829 w/status migrainosus G43821
		intractable: NOS G43839 w/status migrainosus G43831
R0600	**PND: paroxysmal nocturnal dyspnea NOS**	
J64	**Pneumoconiosis unsp**	
		coalworker's J60 asbestois J61
		talc dust J620 silica other than talc J628
		aluminosis J630 bauxite fibrosis J631
		berylliosis J632 graphite fibrosis J633
		siderosis J634 stannosis J635
		d/t other inorganic dust J636
		in tuberculosis J65
J159	**Pneumonia bacterial NOS / If concurrent w/influenza, code flu first**	
J160	**Pneumonia Chlamydial/ If concurrent w/influenza, code flu first**	
J155	**Pneumonia d/t Escherichia coli / If concurrent w/influenza, code flu first**	
J150	**Pneumonia d/t Klebsiella pneumoniae / If concurrent w/influenza, code flu first**	
J157	**Pneumonia d/t Mycoplasma pneumoniae / If concurrent w/influenza, code flu first**	
J151	**Pneumonia d/t Pseudomonas / If concurrent w/influenza, code flu first**	
J1520	**Pneumonia d/t staphylococcus NOS / If concurrent w/influenza, code flu first**	
		staph aureus NOS J15211
		staph aureus methicillin resistant J15212
		other staph J1529
J13	**Pneumonia d/t strep pneumoniae / If concurrent w/influenza, code flu first**	
J153	**Pneumonia d/t streptococcus, group B / If concurrent w/influenza, code flu first**	
		other streptococci J154

J849	**Pneumonia interstitial NOS - first code cause if known / applicable**	

        idiopathic NOS J84111
        desquamative J84117
        lymphoid J842
        endogenous lipoid J8489

J189	**Pneumonia unspecified organism NOS / If concurrent w/influenza, code flu first**

        Bronchopneumonia NOS J180
        Lobar J181 hypostatic J182
        other type unspecified organism J188

J129	**Pneumonia viral NOS**

        adenoviral J120   respiratory synctial virus J121
        parainfluenza J122 Human metapneumovirus J123
        SARS-associated coronavirus J1281
        other viral J1289
        If concurrent w/influenza, code flu first

T148	**PNI: peripheral nerve injury NOS**

        abdomen / lower back / pelvis   S346xx-
        neck S144xx-
        7th character indicates encounter
        A - initial encounter D - subsequent encounter S - sequela

M300	**Polyarteritis nodosa NOS**

        with lung involvement M301   juvenile M302

D45	**Polycythemia vera**
R631	**Polydipsia**
G63	**Polyneuropathy in other diseases NEC**

        Do not separately code polyneuropathy in:
        diabetes, diphtheria, MONO, Lyme disease, mumps,
        postherpetic, rheumatoid arthritis, scleroderma, SLE

G629	**Polyneuropathy NOS**

        inflammatory NOS G619   serum G611
        drug induced G620   alcoholic G621
        radiation induced G6282   critical ilkness G6281
        d/t other toxic agent G622
        chronic inflammatory demyelinating   G6181
        acute postinfective G610   other G6189
        in SLE   M3219   in Lyme disease A6922
        postherpetic B0223   in mumps B2684
        SEQUELAE to toxic polyneuropathy G650
        SEQUELAE to other inflammatory polyneuropathy G651

-	**Polyneuropathy sequelae**

        code first the resulting condition
        to Guillain-Barre' syndrome G650
        to other inflammatory polyneuropathy G651
        to toxic polyneuropathy G652

R632	**Polyphagia**
-	**Polyps colon SEE colon**

R358	**Polyuria NOS**
	frequency of micturition R350
	nocturia R351
	RELATED enlarged prostate N401
E7402	**Pompe disease**
E8020	**Porphyria NOS**
	acute intermittent (hepatic) E8021
	hereditary erythropoietic E800
	cutanea tarda E801
	other E8029
I970	**Postcardiotomy syndrome**
G8383	**Posterior cord syndrome**
K911	**Postgastrectomy syndrome**
I237	**Postinfarction angina**
M963	**Postlaminectomy kyphosis**
M961	**Postlaminectomy syndrome**
F070	**Postleucotomy syndrome**
	Code first underlying physiological condition
I972	**Postmastectomy lymphedema syndrome**
N951	**Postmenopausal climacteric symptoms**
	Includes
	flushing sleeplessness
	lack of concentration headache
N959	**Postmenopausal disorder NOS**
	bleeding / hemorrhage N950
	atrophic vaginitis N952
	climacteric states N951
	other N958
Z79890	**Postmenopausal hormone replacement therapy**
Z780	**Postmenopausal status age related / natural**
I241	**Postmyocardial infarction syndrome**
Z471	**Postop aftercare orthopedic joint replacement**
	Use additional code below to identify the joint -
	shoulder: right Z96611 left Z96612 unsp Z96619
	elbow: right Z96621 left Z96622 unsp Z96629
	wrist: right Z96631 left Z96632 unsp Z96639
	hip: right Z96641 left Z96642 bilat Z96643 unsp Z96649
	knee: right Z96651 left Z96652 bilat Z96653 unsp Z96659
	ankle: right Z96661 left Z96662 unsp Z96669
	finger: right Z96691 left Z96692 bilat Z96693
	other Z96698
T800XX-	**Postop air embolism from infusion / transfusion / injection**
	7th character indicates encounter
	A - initial encounter D - subsequent encounter S - sequela
J95812	**Postop air leak**
H5940	**Postop bleb inflammation/infection NOS (eye)**
	stage 1 H5941
	stage 2 H5942
	stage 3 H5943

K912	**Postop blind loop syndrome**
Z483	**Postop care cancer/neoplasm**
	Also code neoplasm
-	**Postop Care SEE Aftercare also**
T8189X-	**Postop complication NOS**
	7th character indicates encounter
	A - initial encounter D - subsequent encounter S - sequela
Z4803	**Postop drainage change or removal**
R5082	**Postop fever**
T8183X-	**Postop fistula persistent**
	7th character indicates encounter
	A - initial encounter D - subsequent encounter S - sequela
K911	**Postop gastric surgery syndrome**
-	**Postop hematoma / hemorrhage CIRCULATORY system**
	following cardiac catheterization I97610
	following cardiac bypass I97611
	following other circulatory system procedure I97618
	following other procedure I9762
-	**Postop hematoma / hemorrhage DIGESTIVE system**
	following digestive system procedure K91840
	following other procedure K91841
-	**Postop hematoma / hemorrhage EAR & MASTOID PROCESS**
	following procedure on the ear and mastoid process H9541
	following other procedure H9542
-	**Postop hematoma / hemorrhage ENDOCRINE system**
	following an endocrine system procedure E89810
	following other procedure E89811
-	**Postop hematoma / hemorrhage GENITOURINARY system**
	following a genitourinary procedure N99820
	following other procedure N99821
-	**Postop hematoma / hemorrhage MUSCULOSKELETAL system**
	following a musculoskeletal procedure M96830
	following other procedure M96831
-	**Postop hematoma / hemorrhage NERVOUS system**
	following a nervous system procedure G9751
	following other procedure G9752
-	**Postop hematoma / hemorrhage OPHTHALMIC system**
	following an ophthalmic procedure--
	eye & adnexa: right H59311 left H59312
	bilat H59313 unsp H59319
	following other procedure--
	eye & adnexa: right H59321 left H59322
	bilat H59323 unsp H59329
-	**Postop hematoma / hemorrhage RESPIRATORY system**
	following respiratory system procedure J95830
	following other procedure J95831
-	**Postop hematoma / hemorrhage SKIN & SUBCUT system**
	following a dermatologic procedure L7621
	following other procedure L7622

K432	**Postop hernia ventral NOS**
	w/gangrene K431
	incarcerated K430
E891	**Postop hyperglycemia / hypoinsulinemia**
E892	**Postop hypoparathyrodism**
E893	**Postop hypopituitarism**
I9581	**Postop hypotension (not d/t hemodialysis)**
E890	**Postop hypothyroidism**
-	**Postop infarct (cerebrovascular)**
	following cardiac surgery I97820
	following other surgery I97821
T814xx-	**Postop infection NOS any site except OB**
	7th character indicates encounter
	A - initial encounter D - subsequent encounter S - sequela
M6140	**Postop muscle calcification or ossification unsp site**
K912	**Postop nonabsorption NOS**
E8940	**Postop ovary failure asymptomatic**
	symptomatic E8941
-	**Postop pain**
	acute other than thoracotomy G8918
	acute/NOS post thoracotomy G8912
	chronic other than postthoracotomy G8928
	chronic postthoracotomy G8922
J95811	**Postop pneumothorax**
M960	**Postop pseudoarthrosis after fusion or arthrodesis any site**
	Z981 arthrodesis status
K6811	**Postop retroperitoneal abscess**
T888XX-	**Postop seroma except OB**
	7th character indicates encounter
	A - initial encounter D - subsequent encounter S - sequela
T8110x-	**Postop shock NOS**
	cardiogenic T8111x-
	septic T8112x-
	other/ hypovolemic T8119x-
	7th character indicates encounter
	A - initial encounter D - subsequent encounter S - sequela
E895	**Postop testicle hypofunction**
K910	**Postop vomiting after gastrointestinal surgery**
-	**Postop wound aftercare SEE wound care**
F0781	**Posttraumatic brain syndrome non-psychotic**
F4310	**Posttraumatic stress disorder NOS**
	acute F4311 chronic F4312
B960	**PPLO: pleuropneumonia-like organism infection cause of other disease**
	pleuropneumonia-like organism pneumonia J157
I6783	**PRES: posterior reversible encephalopathy syndrome**
-	**Pressure ulcer - SEE site**
I639	**PRIND: prolonged resolving or reversible ischemic neurologic deficit**
	personal history Z8673
K6289	**Proctitis NOS**

K5100	**Proctitis ulcerative chronic unsp**
	w/rectal bleeding K51011
	w/intestinal obstruction K51012
	w/fistula K51013
	w/abscess K51014
	w/other specified complication K51018
	w/unspecified complication K51019
G7111	**PROMM: proximal myotonic myopathy**
N412	**Prostate abscess**
N4289	**Prostate atrophy**
N420	**Prostate calculus / stone**
N421	**Prostate congestion and hemorrhage**
N4283	**Prostate cyst**
N429	**Prostate disorder NOS**
N423	**Prostate dysplasia (PIN I or II)**
N4289	**Prostate fistula/infarction**
N421	**Prostate hemorrhage**
N400	**Prostate hyperplasia/ hypertrophy benign /NOS**
	w/LUTS N401 also code LUTS
-	**Prostate intraepithelial neoplasia**
	type I or II or NOS (histologically confirmed) N423
	type III D075
-	**Prostate neoplasm**
	malignant primary C61
	secondary C7982
	benign D291
	Mets to bone C7951 mets to unsp lymph nodes C779
	Mets to intraabdominal lymph node C772
	Mets to intrapelvic lymph node C775
N402	**Prostate nodular**
	w/LUTS N403 also code LUTS
N4281	**Prostate painful syndrome (prostadynia syndrome)**
R972	**Prostate specific antigen abnormal**
N420	**Prostate stone**
N4289	**Prostate stricture**
I868	**Prostate varices**
A5422	**Prostatitis gonococcal**
N419	**Prostatitis NOS**
	acute N410 chronic N411
	granulomatous N414 other N418
	trichomonal A5902 in actinomycosis N51
	gonococcal: acute A5422 chronic A5422
N413	**Prostatocystitis**
N4282	**Prostatosis syndrome**
Z1611	**PRSA: penicillin resistant staph aureus infection (first code infection) - do not use with MRSA**
	Code may be used to identify any penicillin resistant infection

L299	**Pruritis NOS**	
	genital unsp L293	
	perianal / ani L290	
	senilis L298 scroti L291	
	vulva L292	
R972	**PSA: prostate specific antigen elevated**	
K830	**PSC: primary sclerosing cholangitis**	
M960	**Pseudoarthrosis d/t fusion or arthrodesis**	
K6812	**Psoas muscle abscess**	
L22	**Psoriasiform napkin eruption /erythema /diaper rash**	
L409	**Psoriasis NOS**	
	vulgaris L400 generalized pustular L401	
	guttate L404 pustulosis L403	
	arthropathic unsp L4050	
	distal interphalangeal arthropathy L4051	
	arthritis mutilans L4052	
	spondylitis L4053 juvenile arthropathy L4054	
	other arthropathic L4059	
	other psoriasis L408	
M340	**PSS: progressive systemic sclerosis**	
I471	**PSVT: Paroxysmal supraventricular tachycardia**	
D681	**PTA: plasma thromboplastin antecedent deficiency**	
D67	**PTC: plasma thromboplastin component deficiency**	
D47Z1	**PTLD: post-transplant lymphoproliferative disorder**	
D6951	**PTP: post-transfusion purpura**	
F4310	**PTSD: post traumatic stress disorder NOS**	
	acute F4311 chronic F4312	
R791	**PTT: partial thromboplastin time abnormal**	
K279	**PUD: peptic ulcer disease NOS**	
	SEE PEPTIC ULCER FOR MORE	
J984	**Pulmolithiasis NOS**	
J8402	**Pulmonary alveolar microlithiasis**	
	alveolar proteinosis J8401	
I281	**Pulmonary artery aneurysm NOS**	
I288	**Pulmonary artery arteritis/ endarteritis/ rupture/ stenosis/ stricture**	
J810	**Pulmonary edema acute**	
	chronic / NOS J811	
I2699	**Pulmonary embolism NOS**	
	septic w/acute cor pulmonale I2601	
	w/saddle embolus of pulmonary artery w/cor pulmonale I2602	
	other w/cor pulmonale I2609	
	septic NOS I2690 (code underlying infection first)	
	saddle embolism NOS I2692	
	chronic I2782	
	RELATED	
	personal hx of pulmonary embolism Z86711	
	long term use of anticoagulants Z7901	
J8410	**Pulmonary fibrosis unsp**	

I272	**Pulmonary hypertension NOS**
	pulmonary primary I270
R918	**Pulmonary infiltrate NOS found on imaging**
I379	**Pulmonary valve disorder nonrheumatic unsp**
	stenosis I370 insufficiency I371
	stenosis w/insufficiency I372
	other I378
D692	**Purpura NOS/nonthrombocytopenic NOS/senile**
	allergic/ autoimmune/ rheumatica/ D690
	primary annularis telaniectodes L959
	posttransfusion D6951
	hypergammaglobulinemic D890
	fibrinolytic/fulminans D65
D6949	**Purpura thrombocytopenic primary NOS /other specified**
	hereditary & congenital D6942
	thrombotic M311
I493	**PVC: premature ventricular contractions**
I739	**PVD: peripheral vascular disease NOS**
P912	**PVL: periventricular leukomalacia**
I472	**PVT: paroxysmal ventricular tachycardia**
Q871	**PWS: Prader-Willi syndrome**
N2884	**Pyelitis cystica**
N12	**Pyelonephritis NOS (also pyelitis)**
	acute N10
	chronic nonobstructive reflux associated N110
	chronic obstructive N111
	chronic nonobstructive NOS N118
	chronic NOS N119
	in other diseases N16
	calculous NOS N209
N2885	**Pyeloureteritis cystica**
K311	**Pyloric obstruction/stenosis acquired**
K313	**Pylorospasm NEC**
K2960	**Pylorus erosion**
	w/hemorrhage K2961
L080	**Pyoderma NOS any site**
	gangrenous L88
	vegetans L0881
G8250	**Quadriplegia NOS**
	complete C1-C4 G8251 C5-C7 G8253
	incomplete C1-C4 G8252 C5-C7 G8254
M069	**RA: rheumatoid arthritis (except spine or juvenile) NOS**
N3040	**Radiation RELATED cystitis**
	w/hematuria N3041
Z5189	**Radiation therapy convalescence**

M5410	**Radiculopathy unsp**	
	occipito-atlanto-axial M5411	
	cervical M5412	
	cervicothoracic M5413	
	thoracic M5414	
	thoracolumbar M5415	
	lumbar M5416	
	lumbosacral M5417	
	sacral and sacrococcygeal M5418	
D4620	**RAEB: refractory anemia with excess blasts NOS**	
	RAEB-1: refractory anemia with excess blasts-1 D4621	
	RAEB-2: refractory anemia with excess blasts-2 D4622	
D461	**RARS: refractory anemia with ring sideroblasts**	
R21	**Rash NOS**	
	diaper L22 heat L740	
	drug induced: generalized L270 localized L271	
	food induced L272	
M0500	**RASK: rheumatoid arthritis with splenomegaly and leukopenia NOS**	
	aka Felty's syndrome	
A259	**Rat bite fevers NOS**	
	spirillosis (Sodokui) A250	
	streptobacillosis A251	
I7300	**Raynaud's syndrome NOS**	
	w/gangrene I7301	
I4510	**RBBB: right bundle branch block NOS**	
	other I4519	
	SEE Heart block for more	
D46A	**RCMD: refractory cytopenia with multilineage dysplasia**	
	w/ ring sideroblasts (RCMD RS) D46B	
J80	**RDS: respiratory distress syndrome acute NOS**	
K611	**Rectal abscess / cellulitis**	
K604	**Rectal fistula**	
N816	**Rectocele female**	
	male K623	
K6289	**Rectum cyst NOS**	
N805	**Rectum endometriosis**	
K602	**Rectum fissure**	
K603	**Rectum fistula**	
A546	**Rectum gonorrhea**	
K6289	**Rectum granuloma/ irritation NOS**	
K625	**Rectum hemorrhage**	
A563	**Rectum infection d/T chlamydia trachomatis**	
-	**Rectum neoplasm**	
	malignant primary C20	
	secondary C785	
	benign D128	
	Mets to bone C7951 mets to unsp lymph nodes C779	
	Mets to intraabdominal lymph node C772	
	Mets to intrapelvic lymph node C775	

K621	**Rectum polyp NOS**
	adenomatous D128
K623	**Rectum prolapse except hemorrhoids**
K644	**Rectum skin tags**
K624	**Rectum stenosis/stricture**
K626	**Rectum ulcer NOS/ solitary/ stercoral**
I722	**Renal artery aneurysm**
I701	**Renal artery atherosclerosis**
I7773	**Renal artery dissection**
N289	**Renal insufficiency acute**
	chronic N189
N269	**Renal sclerosis NOS**
Z1610	**Resistance to antibiotics beta lactam type NOS**
	penicillins Z1611
	Extended spectrum beta lactamase Z1612
	other Z1619
Z1620	**Resistance to antibiotics NOS**
	vancomycin Z1621
	vancomycin related Z1622
	quinolones / fluoroquinilones Z1623
	multiple Z1624 other Z1629
Z9911	**Respirator dependence**
J398	**Respiratory disease upper tract NOS**
J80	**Respiratory distress acute**
-	**Respiratory failure**
	acute: NOS J9600 w/hypoxia J9601 w/hypercapnia J9602
	chronic: NOS J9610 w/hypoxia J9611 w/hypercapnia J9612
	unsp: NOS J9690 w/hypoxia J9691 w/hypercapnis J9692
	acute and chronic:
	NOS J9620 w/hypoxia J9621 w/hypercapnia J9622
	postop acute J95821 postop acute with chronic J95822
M3130	**Respiratory granulomatosis necrotizing NOS**
	w/renal involvement M3131
J393	**Respiratory hypersensitivity reaction NOS**
J069	**Respiratory infection upper acute NOS (URI)**
-	**Respiratory pain**
	on respiration R071
	precordial pain R072
	pleurodynia R0781
	intercostal pain R0782
	anterior chest wall pain R0789
G2581	**Restless legs syndrome**
-	**Retina hemorrhage**
	unsp H3560 bilateral H3563
	right H3561 left H3562

G937	**Reyes syndrome**
	RELATED adverse effect of aspirin T39015-
	RELATED adverse effect of other salicylates T39095-
	for RELATED 7th character indicates encounter
	A - initial encounter D - subsequent encounter S - sequela
D569	**RGM: Rietti-Greppi-Micheli anemia**
I099	**RHD: rheumatic heart disease NOS**
	acute unsp I019 with chorea I020
J309	**Rhinitis allergic NOS**
	d/t pollen J301 other seasonal J302
	d/t food J305 d/t animal hair J3081
	other J3089 vasomotor J300
J310	**Rhinitis chronic**
	RELATED CODES
	tobacco use Z720
	history of tobacco use Z87891
	Nicotine dependence NOS F17200
	exposure to environmental tobacco smoke Z7722
	occupational exposure to environmental tobacco smoke Z5731
E550	**Rickets active, d/t vitamin D deficiency**
K4090	**RIH: right inguinal hernia SEE INGUINAL HERNIA FOR MORE**
I639	**RIND: reversible ischemic neurological deficit**
	RIND-hx personal history Z8673
H35179	**RLF: retrolental fibroplasia NOS**
	right H35171 left H35172 bilateral H35173
G2581	**RLS: restless legs syndrome**
L719	**Rosacea unsp**
-	**Rotator cuff syndrome (nontraumatic)**
	complete: unsp M75120 right M75121 left M75122
	incomplete: unsp M75110 right M75111 Left M75112
	unspecified: unsp M75100 right M75101 left M75102
B779	**Roundworm unsp**
	w/intestinal complications B770
	w/pneumonia B7781
	w/other complication B7789
B974	**RSV: respiratory synctial virus infection as cause of other disease**
	respiratory synctial virus pneumonia J121
B069	**Rubella NOS**
	w/ neurological complication unsp B0600
	encephalitis B0601 meningitis B0602
	w/other neuro complications B0609
	pneumonia B0681 arthritis B0682
	other complications B0689
I823	**RVT: renal vein thrombosis**
S332	**Sacroiliac dislocation**
	7th character indicates encounter
	A= initial encounter D=subsequent S=sequela

S336	**Sacroiliac sprain**
	7th character indicates encounter
	A= initial encounter D=subsequent S=sequela
M461	**Sacroiliitis NOS**
L89159	**Sacrum pressure ulcer NOS**
	unstageable L89150
	stage 1 L89151 stage 2 L89152
	stage 3 L89153 stage 4 L89154
A029	**Salmonella infection NOS**
	localized NOS A0220 meningitis A0221
	pneumonia A0222 arthritis A0223
	osteomyelitis A0224 pyelonephritis A0225
	sepsis A021 enteritis A020 other A028
A5429	**Salpingitis gonococcal**
N7091	**Salpingitis unsp**
	Chronic N7011
	Acute N7001
N834	**Salpingocele**
D869	**Sarcoidosis NOS**
	lung D860 lymph nodes D861 lung & lymph nodes D862
	skin D863 meningitis D8681 myocarditis D8685
	multiple cranial nerve palsies D8682
	pyelonephritis D8684 arthropathy D8686
	myositis D8687 other sites D8689
B9721	**SARS-severe acute respiratory syndrome, coronavirus infection**
	Above code is used for "as cause of other disease"
	pneumonia d/t J1281 acute URI J069
	exposure to Z2089
	observation for suspected exposure Z2001
	coronavirus infection unsp B342
I339	**SBE: subacute bacterial endocarditis**
	infective I330
K5660	**SBO: small bowel obstruction NOS**
	postoperative K913
K912	**SBS: short bowel syndrome**
F458	**SBS: shy bladder syndrome**
I2542	**SCAD: spontaneous coronary artery dissection**
D571	**SCD: sickle-cell disease NOS**
	w/unsp crisis D5700 & thalassemia D57419
	w/acute chest syndrome D5701 & thalassemia D57411
	w/ splenic sequestration D5702 & thalassemia D57412
	sickle-cell thalassemia NOS D5740
Z8241	**SCD: sudden cardiac death family history**

F209	**Schizophrenia NOS**
	paranoid F200
	disorganized F201
	catatonic F202
	undifferentiated / atypical F203
	residual F205
	schizophreniform psychosis F2081
	other F2089
	cyclic F250
G5700	**Sciatic nerve lesion NOS**
	right G5701 left G5702
M5430	**Sciatica unsp**
	right M5431 left M5432
	w/lumbago: unsp M5440 right M5441 left M5442
D819	**SCID: severe combined immunodeficiency NOS**
	w/ reticular dysgenesis D810
	w/ low T and B cell numbers D811
	ww/ low or normal B cell numbers D812
M419	**Scoliosis NOS any level**
	d/t radiation NOS M965
	idiopathic infantile NOS M4100
	idiopathic NOS M4120
	thoracogenic NOS M4130
E54	**Scurvy**
A419	**Sepsis / septicemia NOS**
A4150	**Sepsis d/t gram negative organisms NOS**
	d/t E. coli A4151
	d/t Pseudomonas A4152
	d/t Serratia A4153
	other gram negative sepsis A4159
A413	**Sepsis d/t Hemophilus influenzae**
A4101	**Sepsis d/t staph aureus NOS**
	Methicillin resistant A4102 (MRSA)
A412	**Sepsis d/t staph NOS**
A409	**Sepsis d/t strep unsp**
	group A A400 group B A401
	s. pneumoniae A403 other A408
	Use after cause code such as
	postop strep sepsis T814xx-
	infection following immunization T880xx-
	local d/t IV T80212- bloodstream d/t IV T80211-
	other d/t IV T80218- unsp d/t IV T80219-
	for T codes, 7th character indicates encounter
	A - initial encounter D - subsequent encounter S - sequela

T814	**Sepsis postprocedure also code organism if known**
	post immunization T880xx-
	7th character indicates encounter
	A - initial encounter D - subsequent encounter S - sequela
	blood infection d/t IV T80211
	RELATED if applicable Severe sepsis R6520
R6520	**Sepsis severe NOS**
	w/septic shock R6521
	RELATED
	critical illness: myopathy G7281 polyneuropathy G6281
	disseminated intravascular coagulopathy D65
	septic encephalopathy G9341
	sepsis NOS A419 bloodstream infection d/t IV T80211-
	postop infection T814xx-
	For T codes above, 7th character indicates encounter
	A - initial encounter D - subsequent encounter S - sequela
	acute kidney failure N179 SEE kidney failure for more
-	**Sezary disease**
	unsp site C8410 head/face/neck C8411 intrathoracic C8412
	intra-abdominal C8413 axilla / arm C8414 inguinal / leg C8415
	intrapelvic C8416 spleen C8417 multiple C8418 extranodal C8419
A039	**Shigellosis NOS**
	d/t Shigella d/t Shigella dysenteriae A030
	d/t Shigella flexneri A031
	d/t Shigella boydii A032
	d/t Shigella sonnei A033
	d/t other A038
Z9989	**Shigellosis unspecified**
B029	**Shingles NOS**
	for specified complications see herpes zoster
T782XX-	**Shock anaphylactic NOS**
	reaction to food unsp T7800x- d/t peanuts T7801x-
	d/t shellfish T7802x- d/t eggs T7808x-
	d/t blood / blood products T8051x-
	d/t vaccination T8052x- d/t other serum T8059x-
	as adverse effect of medicine T886xx-
	7th character indicates encounter
	A - initial encounter D - subsequent encounter S - sequela
R579	**Shock NOS**
	cardiogenic R570
	hypovolemic R571
	other R578
-	**Shock postop SEE Postop shock**
K912	**Short bowel syndrome**
M24619	**Shoulder ankylosis NOS**
	right M24611 left M24612

- **Shoulder bone cyst**
    solitary cyst: unsp M85419 right M85411 left M85412
    aneurysmal cyst: change 4th character to 5
    other cyst: change 4th character to 6
- **Shoulder bursitis**
    unsp M7550 right M7551 left M7552
- **Shoulder capsulitis adhesive**
    unsp M7500 right M7501 left M7502

M94219 **Shoulder chondromalacia unsp**
    right M94211 left M94212

M24519 **Shoulder contractures unsp**
    right M24511 left M24512

M24319 **Shoulder dislocation pathological NOS unsp**
    right M24311 left M24312

M24419 **Shoulder dislocation recurrent unsp**
    right M24411 left M24412

M25419 **Shoulder effusion (joint) unsp**
    right M25411 left M25412

- **Shoulder fracture pathological NOS / (in neoplastic disease below)**
    unsp M84419- right M84411- left M84412-
    7th character indicates encounter/status
    A - initial   S - sequela
    D - subsequent routine healing
    G - subsequent delayed healing
    K - subsequent nonunion   P - subsequent malunion
    Change 4th character to 5 for 'in neoplastic disease'
- **Shoulder gout chronic**
    idiopathic/primary right M1A011- left M1A012- unsp M1A019-
    lead induced right M1A111- left M1A112- unsp M1A119-
    drug induced right M1A211- left M1A212- unsp M1A219-
    d/t renal impairment right M1A311- left M1A312- unsp M1A319-
    other secondary right M1A411- left M1A412- unsp M1A419-
    The appropriate 7th character
    0 = without tophus (tophi) 1 = with tophus (tophi)

M25019 **Shoulder hemarthrosis unsp**
    right M25011 left M25012

- **Shoulder impingement syndrome**
    unsp M7540 right M7541 left M7542

M24819 **Shoulder joint instability NOS unsp**
    right M24811 left M24812

M24019 **Shoulder joint mice unsp**
    right M24011 left M24012

M19019 **Shoulder osteoarthritis primary unsp**
    right M19011 left M19012

M80019-	**Shoulder osteoporosis age related w/current fracture unsp**
	right M80011- left M80012-
	7th character indicates encounter/status
	A - initial D - subsequent routine healing
	G - subsequent delayed healing S - sequela
	K - subsequent nonunion P - subsequent malunion
M25519	**Shoulder pain (joint) unsp**
	right M25511 left M25512
-	**Shoulder rotator cuff rupture non-traumatic**
	unsp M75120 right M75121 left M75122
-	**Shoulder rotator cuff syndrome**
	NOS: unsp M75100 right M75101 left M75102
	incomplete: unsp M75110 right M75111 left M75112
	complete: unsp M75120 right M75121 left M75122
M25619	**Shoulder stiffness of joint NOS unsp**
	right M25611 left M25612
-	**Shoulder tendinitis calcifying**
	unsp M7530 right M7531 left M7532
G2583	**Shuddering benign attacks**
D571	**Sickle-cell disease NOS**
	w/unsp crisis D5700 & thalassemia D57419
	w/acute chest syndrome D5701 & thalassemia D57411
	w/ splenic sequestration D5702 & thalassemia D57412
	sickle-cell thalassemia NOS D5740
-	**Sinusitis ACUTE**
	unsp J0190 unsp recurrent J0191
	maxillary: unsp J0100 recurrent J0101
	frontal: unsp J0110 recurrent J0111
	ethmoidal: unsp J0120 recurrent J0121
	sphenoidal: unsp J0130 recurrent J0131
	pansinusitus: unsp J0140 recurrent J0141
	other: unsp J0180 recurrent J0181
J329	**Sinusitis chronic NOS**
	maxillary J320 frontal J321
	ethmoidal J322 sphenoidal J323
	pansinusitis J324 other J328
-	**SIRS common underlying infections, code before SIRS**
	dt venous cath: local T80212- bloodstream T80211-
	other T80218- NOS T80219-
	d/t transfusion/infusion/injection: blood products T8022x- other T8029x-
	d/t procedure T814xx-
	For "T" codes, 7th character indicates encounter
	A - initial encounter D - subsequent encounter S - sequela
	sepsis: NOS A419 d/t e coli A4151 d/t pseudomonas A4152
	d/t gram negative NOS A4150 d/t enterrococcus A4181
	d/t MSSA A4101 d/t MRSA A4102 d/t serratia A4153
	d/t unsp staph A412 d/t hemophilus influenzae A413

-	**SIRS organ dysfunction common RELATED codes**	
	acute respiratory failure NOS J9600 w/hypoxia J9601	
	w/hypercapnia J9602	
	myopathy G7281 polyneuropathy G6281	
	acute kidney failure: NOS N179 w/tubular necrosis N170	
	w/cortical necrosis N171 w/medullary necrosis N172	
	encephalopathy G9341 DIC D65	
-	**SIRS: systemic inflammatory response syndrome non-infectious NOS**	
	noninfectious: NOS R6510 w/ acute organ dysfunction R6511	
	INFECTIOUS R6520 w/septic shock R6521	
	Code underlying cause / infection first	
-	**SIS: subacromial impingement syndrome NOS**	
	unsp M7540 right M7541 left M7542	
L513	**SJS-TEN: Stevens-Johnson syndrome toxic epidermal necrolysis overlap syndrome**	
	just SJS L511	
R239	**Skin changes NOS**	
	desquamation/induration/scaling R234	
	petechiae R233	
	clammy R231	
L729	**Skin cyst follicular unsp**	
	epidermal L720	
	pilar L7211	
	trichodermal L7212	
	sebaceous L723	
	other L728	
R229	**Skin lump/mass/swelling NOS**	
	head R220 neck R221 trunk R222	
S43439-	**SLAP: superior glenoid labrum lesions NOS**	
	right S43431- left S43432-	
	7th character indicates encounter	
	A - initial encounter D - subsequent encounter S - sequela	
M329	**SLE: Lupus erythematosus systemic NOS**	
	Drug induced M320 w/lung involvement M3213	
	w/endocarditis M3211 w/pericarditis M3212	
	w/tubulo-interstitial disease M3215	
	w/glomerular disease M3214	
	w/other organ or system involvement M3219	
	other forms of SLE M328	
G4730	**Sleep apnea NOS code first any underlying condition**	
	primary central G4731	
	obstructive G4733	
	in other conditions G4737	
	other specified G4739	
G3182	**SNE: subacute necrotizing encephalopathy**	
R0602	**SOB: short of breath**	
R900	**SOL: space occupying lesion intracranial**	
J029	**Sore throat acute**	
	chronic J312	

-	**Spinal puncture complication**
	cerebrospinal fluid leak G970
	headache G971
	hemorrhage/hematoma G9751
M4800	**Spine stenosis / caudal stenosis unsp**
	occipito-atlanto-axial M4801
	cervical M4802
	cervicothoracic M4803
	thoracic M4804
	thoracolumbar M4805
	lumbar M4806
	lumbosacral M4807
	sacral and sacrococcygeal M4808
-	**Spleen disorders**
	atrophy D730 hypersplenism D731
	chronic congestive splenomegaly D732
	abscess D733 cyst D734
	infarction / rupture / torsion D735
	neutropenic splenomegaly D7381
	fibrosis / splenitis NOS D7389
	unspecified D739
	splenomegaly NOS R161
C261	**Spleen fibrosarcoma**
R948	**Spleen function test abnormal NOS**
-	**Spleen neoplasm**
	malignant primary C261
	secondary C7889
	benign D139
	Mets to bone C7951 mets to unsp lymph nodes C779
	Mets to intraabdominal lymph node C772
R161	**Splenomegaly NOS**
	neutropenic D7381
	chronic congestive D732
A0819	**SRV: small round virus NOS infection of intestine (enteritis, gastroenteropathy)**
A811	**SSPE: subacute sclerosing panencephalitis**
I495	**SSS: sick sinus syndrome**
L00	**SSS: staphylococcal scalded skin syndrome (also SSSS)**
B958	**Staphylococcus infection NOS as cause of disease**
	specified other than aureus B957
K7581	**Steatohepatitis nonalcoholic**
B9623	**STEC: shiga toxin producing e coli NOS**
	STEC 0157 B9621 other STEC not 0157 B9622
I213	**STEMI: ST elevation myocardial infarction NOS**
	SEE myocardial infarction ST elevated for more
G2582	**Stiff-man syndrome**
R413	**STM: short term memory (loss)**
-	**Stoma infection SEE type, eg colostomy, tracheostomy**
K31819	**Stomach and duodenum angiodysplasia**
	w/bleeding K31811

K3189	**Stomach congestion passive**
K3182	**Stomach dieulafoy lesion hemorrhagic**
K310	**Stomach dilatation/distention acute**
-	**Stomach neoplasm**

        MALIGNANT Primary
        body C162   cardia C160
        pyloric antrum C163   pylorus C164
        lesser curvature C165   unspecified C169
        greater curvature C166 fundus C161
        overlapping sites C168
        Malignant secondary all sites C7889
        Benign all sites D131
        Mets to bone   C7951   mets to unsp lymph nodes C779
        Mets to intraabdominal lymph node C772

K312	**Stomach stenosis/stricture hourglass type non congenital**
-	**STOMACH ULCER -- SEE gastric**
K289	**Stomal ulcer unsp NOS**

      acute: NOS K283 w/hemorrhage K280 w/perforation K281
      acute: w/both hemorrhage & perforation K282
      chronic / unsp: NOS K287 w/hemorrhage K284
      chronic / unsp: w/perforation: K285
      chronic / unsp: w/both hemorrhage & perforation K286

A690	**Stomatitis acute necrotizing ulcerative (Vincent's)(gangrenous)**

        Necrotizing ulcerative (acute) gingivostomatitis A691

B0861	**Stomatitis bovine**
B088	**Stomatitis epizootic**
B002	**Stomatitis herpetic**
R195	**Stool abnormality bulky/ color/ fat/ mucus/ occult blood/ pus**
K921	**Stools black (melana) - do not use w/ulcer**
J020	**Strep throat pharyngitis**
B955	**Streptococcus infection NOS as cause of disease**

        group A B950 group B B951
        group C B954   group G B954
        group D (enterococcus) B952
        s. pneumoniae B953

I639	**Stroke SEE Cerebral infarction for more**
R401	**Stupor (semi-coma)**
G44059	**SUNCT: short lasting unilateral neuralgiform headache with conjunctival injection and tearing NOS**

        intractable G44051

I871	**SVCS: superior vena cava syndrome**
I471	**SVT: supraventricular tachycardia**
-	**SWALLOWING DIFFICULTY - SEE Dysphagia**
R55	**Syncope and collapse NOS**
G44099	**TAC: trigeminal autonomic cephalgia NEC NOS**

        intractable G44091

R000	**Tachycardia NOS**
	nonparoxysmal I4589
	paroxysmal atrial I471
	paroxysmal essential I479
	paroxysmal ventricular I472
I495	**Tachycardia-bradycardia syndrome**
R0682	**Tachypnea**
E8771	**TACO: transfusion associated circulatory overload**
I7101	**TAD: thoracic aorta dissection**
B681	**Taenia saginata**
B680	**Taenia solium intestinal form (cysticercosis)**
	larval NOS B699 eye B691
	myositis B6981 other sites B6989
	central nervous system B690
B719	**Tapeworm NOS**
	beef B681 pork B680 pork larva NOS B699
	dog B711 rat / dwarf B710 fish B700
Q262	**TAPVR: total anomalous pulmonary venous return**
Q872	**TAR: thrombocytopenia w/absent radius syndrome**
G5750	**Tarsal tunnel syndrome NOS**
	right G5751 left G5752
E7502	**Tay-Sachs disease**
A159	**TB: tuberculosis respiratory NOS**
	respiratory primary A157 lung A150
	larynx trachea bronchus A155
	intrathoracic lymph nodes A154
	other respiratory A158 pleurisy A156
I495	**TBS: tachycardia bradycardia syndrome**
J860	**TEF: tracheoesophageal fistula**
	following tracheostomy J9504
M89160	**TEGD: tibial epiphyseal growth disturbance COMPLETE right proximal**
	left proximal M89161 right distal M89164 left distal M89165
M89162	**TEGD: tibial epiphyseal growth disturbance PARTIAL right proximal**
	left proximal M89163
	right distal M89166 left distal M89167
M2660	**Temporomandibular joint disorder unsp**
	adhesions/ankylosis M2661
	pain M2662
	articular disc disorder M2663
	other spec disorder of TMJ M2669
Z515	**Terminal care**
N454	**Testicle abscess**
N501	**Testicle hematoma**
N433	**Testicle hydrocele NOS**
	encysted N430
	infected N431
	other N432
E291	**Testicle hypofunction NOS**
	postop E895

A5619	Testicle infection d/t chlamydia trachomatis
A35	**Tetanus NOS**
C710	**Thalamus neoplasm malignant primary**
	Secondary C7931 Benign D330
	Mets to bone C7951
	mets to esophageal nodes C771
L97129	**Thigh ulcer non-pressure chronic left NOS**
	limited to skin L97121
	w/fat layer exposed L97122
	w/muscle necrosis L97123
	w/bone necrosis L97124
L97119	**Thigh ulcer non-pressure chronic right NOS**
	limited to skin L97111
	w/fat layer exposed L97112
	w/muscle necrosis L97113
	w/bone necrosis L97114
L97109	**Thigh ulcer non-pressure chronic unspecified side NOS**
	limited to skin L97101
	w/fat layer exposed L97102
	w/muscle necrosis L97103
	w/bone necrosis L97104
-	Thoracic neuritis or radiculitis NOS - SEE Radiculopathy
C140	**Throat neoplasm malignant primary**
	Secondary C7989 Benign D109
	Mets to bone C7951 mets to esophageal nodes C771
	Mets to axilla / arm lymph node C773
	Mets to cervical lymph node C770
J029	**Throat sore acute NOS**
	chronic J312
D696	**Thrombocytopenia unsp**
	primary NOS D6949
	heparin induced D7582
E329	**Thymus disease unsp**
	persistent hyperplasia / hypertrophy E320
	abscess E321
	other E328
	aplasia or hypoplasia w/ immunodeficiency D821
E060	**Thyroid abscess**
E034	**Thyroid atrophy acquired**
-	**THYROID CRISIS OR STORM -- SEE thyrotoxicosis**
E041	**Thyroid cyst**
E039	**Thyroid deficit NOS**
	d/t iodine / PAS/ iatrogenic E032
	secondary acquired NOS E038
	postop or d/t radiation therapy E890
	congenital E009
E079	**Thyroid disorder NOS**
E049	**Thyroid enlargement NOS**
R946	**Thyroid function test abnormal NOS**

E0789	**Thyroid hemorrhage/infarction**
B6731	**Thyroid infection Echinococcus granulosus**
-	**THYROID INSUFFICIENCY -- SEE hypothyroidism**
E041	**Thyroid nodule NOS nontoxic**
E069	**Thyroiditis NOS**
	acute/pyogenic E060
	chronic: NOS / fibrous E065
	autoimmune / Hashimoto's E063
	de Quervain's / subacute E061
	drug induced E064
	chronic w/transient thyrotoxicosis E062
E0590	**Thyrotoxicosis NOS**
	w/goiter toxic nodular: NOS E0520 w/crisis E0521
	w/goiter uninodular: E0510 w/crisis E0511
	w/goiter toxic diffuse: E0500 w/crisis E0501
	factitia/ d/t overproduction of TSH: E0540 w/crisis E0541
	d/t ectopic thyroid nodule: E0530 w/crisis E0531
	NOS w/crisis E0591
	RELATED Cardiomyopathy I43
	RELATED Eaton-Lambert Syndrome/ Myasthenia G733
	RELATED myopathy G737
G459	**TIA: transient ischemic attack**
F959	**Tic NOS**
	drug induced G2561
	Tic douloureux G500
	chronic motor or vocal F951
	Tourette's F952
	transient F950
	other of organic origin G2569 other F958
B359	**Tinea microsporic NOS**
	blanca B362 nigra B361
	imbricata B355 manuum B352
	pedis B353 unguium B351
	capitis B350 cruris B356
	flava/versicolor B360
	corporis B354
M2660	**TMJ: temporomandibular joint - disorder NOS**
	adhesions/ankylosis M2661
	pain M2662
	articular disc disorder M2663
	other spec disorder of TMJ M2669
N7093	**TOA: tubo-ovarian abscess NOS salpingitis and oophoritis unsp**
	salpingitis NOS alone N7091 oophoritis NOS alone N7092
L03039	**Toe cellulitis unsp**
	right L03031 left L03032

- **Toe gout acute/NOS (and foot / ankle)**
    idiopathic/primary right M10071 left M10072 unsp M10079
    lead induced right M10171 left M10172 unsp M10179
    drug induced right M10271 left M10272 unsp M10279
    d/t renal impairment right M10371 left M10372 unsp M10379
    other secondary right M10471 left M10472 unsp M10479
- **Toe gout chronic**
    idiopathic/primary right M1A071- left M1A072- unsp M1A079-
    lead induced right M1A171- left M1A172- unsp M1A179-
    drug induced right M1A271- left M1A272- unsp M1A279-
    d/t renal impairment right M1A371- left M1A372- unsp M1A379-
    other secondary right M1A471- left M1A472- unsp M1A479-
    The appropriate 7th character
    0 = without tophus (tophi) 1 = with tophus (tophi)
- **Toes fracture pathological NOS / (in neoplastic disease below)**
    unsp M84479- right M84477- left M84478-
    7th character indicates encounter/status
    A - initial S - sequela
    D - subsequent routine healing
    G - subsequent delayed healing
    K - subsequent nonunion P - subsequent malunion
    Change 4th character to 5 for 'in neoplastic disease'

J0390	**Tonsillitis acute NOS**

    acute NOS recurrent J0391
    strep acute: NOS J0300 recurrent J0301
    d/t other spec organism: NOS J0380 recurrent J0381

M436	**Torticollis NOS**

    ocular R29891 hysterical F444
    psychogenic F458 spasmodic G243
    traumatic recurrent S134

G540	**TOS: thoracic outlet syndrome**
M358	**Toxic oil syndrome**
A483	**Toxic shock syndrome**
C33	**Trachea neoplasm malignant primary**

    secondary C7839   benign D142
    RELATED codes
    exposure to environmental tobacco smoke Z7722
    history of tobacco use Z87891
    occupational exposure to environmental tobacco smoke Z5731
    tobacco use Z720
    Mets to bone   C7951   mets to unsp lymph nodes C779
    Mets to axilla / arm lymph node   C773

J0410	**Tracheitis acute NOS**

    w/obstruction J0411

Z430	**Tracheostomy care / aftercare**

    status w/o need for care Z930

J9500	**Tracheostomy complication NOS**
	stoma hemorrhage J9501 other J9509
	tracheo-esophageal fistula J9504
	malfunction J9503 stoma infection J9502
	For stoma infection code also code type of infection:
	eg. neck cellulitis L038 or a sepsis code
A719	**Trachoma unsp**
	initial stage A710
	active stage A711
J9584	**TRALI: transfusion related acute lung injury**
-	**Transfusion reaction hemolytic (blood)**
	acute d/t Rh incompatibility T80410-
	acute d/t ABO incompatibility T80310-
	delayed 24 hr+ d/t Rh incompatibility T80411-
	delayed 24 hr+ d/t ABO incompatibility T80311-
	unsp d/t Rh incompatibility T80419-
	unsp d/t ABO incompatibility T80319-
	7th character indicates encounter
	A - initial encounter D - subsequent encounter S - sequela
-	**Transfusion reaction NON hemolytic (blood)**
	ABO incompatibility unsp T8030x-
	AB0 incompatibility other spec T8039x-
	Rh incompatibility unsp T8040x-
	Rh incompatibility other spec T8049x-
	7th character indicates encounter
	A - initial encounter D - subsequent encounter S - sequela
R251	**Tremor NOS**
	essential / familial G250
	hysterical F444
	intention/ other G252
	drug induced G251
A599	**Trichomoniasis NOS**
	intestinal A078 prostatitis A5902
	urethritis A5903 urogenital NOS A5900
	vulvovaginitis A5901
	other specified urogenital A5909
	specified site other A598
I369	**Tricuspid valve disorder nonrheumatic unsp**
	stenosis I360 insufficiency I361
	stenosis w/insufficiency I362
	other I368
G509	**Trigeminal nerve disorder NOS**
	neuralgia G500
	atypical face pain G501
-	**Trypanosomiasis American SEE Chaga's disease**
E0580	**TSH: thyroid stimulating hormone overproduction NOS**
	with crisis/storm E0581
A483	**TSS: toxic shock syndrome (also code organism)**
M311	**TTP: thrombotic thrombocytopenic purpura**

-	**Tuberculosis respiratory / genitourinary NOS**
	NOS A159 respiratory primary A157 lung A150
	larynx trachea bronchus A155
	intrathoracic lymph nodes A154
	other respiratory A158 pleurisy A156
	GU system NOS A1810 kidney & ureter A1811
	bladder A1812 prostate A1814 cervix A1816
	female pelvic inflammatory disease A1817
	vulva A1818 testicles A1816
A219	**Tularemia unsp**
	ulceroglandular A210 oculoglandular A211
	pulmonary A212 gastrointestinal A213
	generalized A217 other A218
-	**UCPPS: urologic chronic pelvic pain syndrome -**
	No specific code. If term is used, clarify with physician.
	possible codes -
	female interstitial cystitis: N3010 w/ hematuria N3011
	male chronic prostatitis N411
-	**UIH: unilateral inguinal hernia SEE Inguinal hernia**
-	**Ulcer GI peptic SEE Peptic**
N19	**Uremia NOS**
	chronic N189 extrarenal R392
D593	**Uremic syndrome hemolytic**
	RELATED pneumococcal pneumonia J13
	RELATED shigella dyenteriae A039
	RELATED e colli infection B962- final character below
	NOS 0 STEC 0157 1 other spec STEC 2
	other unsp STEC 3 non STEC 9
N2889	**Ureter adhesions**
N135	**Ureter angulation/constriction including postop**
N201	**Ureter calculus**
	w/calculus of kidney N202
R934	**Ureter filling defect (found on imaging)**
N2889	**Ureter fistula**
N201	**Ureter obstruction due to stone**
N2889	**Ureter polyp**
N2889	**Ureter prolapse**
	obstructed N135
	infected N136
N2886	**Ureteritis cystica**
N2889	**Ureterocele**
N340	**Urethra abscess**
N368	**Urethra colic/ cyst/ granuloma**
N360	**Urethra fistula**
N3641	**Urethra hypermobility**
N368	**Urethra instability**
N3642	**Urethra intrinsic sphincter deficiency**
N362	**Urethra polyp**
N368	**Urethra prolapse / rupture nontraumatic**

N359	**Urethra stricture NOS**	
	other NEC N358	
-	**Urethra stricture post-traumatic FEMALE**	
	d/t childbirth N35021 other N35028	
-	**Urethra stricture post-traumatic MALE**	
	meatal N35010 bulbous N35011	
	membranous N35012 anterior N35013	
	NOS N35014	
N3512	**Urethra stricture postinfective NOS female**	
N35119	**Urethra stricture postinfective NOS male**	
	meatal N35111 bulbous N35112	
	membranous N35113 anterior N35114	
N9912	**Urethra stricture postop FEMALE**	
N99114	**Urethra stricture postop unsp MALE**	
	meatal N99110 bulbous N99111	
	membranous N99112 anterior N991113	
N342	**Urethra ulcer**	
N320	**Urethral contracture/ obstruction/ stenosis**	
T83098-	**Urethral catheter indwelling mechanical complication other**	
	includes obstruction/perforation/protrusion	
	leakage T83038- displacement T83028-	
	mechanical breakdown T83018-	
	7th character indicates encounter -	
	A - initial encounter D - subsequent encounter S - sequela	
R369	**Urethral discharge NOS**	
	specified w/o blood R360	
	w/blood R361	
N343	**Urethral syndrome unspecified**	
N341	**Urethritis infectious nonspecific**	
	trichomonal A5903	
	gonococcal A5401	
	chlamydia trachomatis A5601	
	candidal B3741	
N342	**Urethritis NOS**	
	nonspecific / nongonococcal N341	
N342	**Urethritis postmenopausal**	
N810	**Urethrocele female**	
N360	**Urethrorectal fistula**	
R369	**Urethrorrhea NOS**	
	w/o blood R360	
	hematospermia R361	
N3030	**Urethrotrigonitis NOS**	
	w/ hematuria N3031	
N322	**Urethrovesical fistula**	
J069	**URI: upper respiratory infection acute NOD**	

N209	**Urinary calculus NOS**
	lower tract NOS N219
	lower tract spec not bladder N218
	in urethra N211
	in bladder N210
	in kidney N200
	in ureter N201
	kidney & ureter N202
T8351x-	**Urinary catheter infected / inflammed**
	7th character indicates encounter
	A - initial encounter D - subsequent encounter S - sequela
N360	**Urinary fistula NOS**
-	**Urinary incontinence**
	stress N393 urge N3941
	w/o sensory awareness N3942
	post-void dribbling N3943 overflow N39490
	nocturnal enuresis N3944 continuous leakage N3945
	mixed urge and stress N3946
	urinary incontinence other / reflex / total N39498
N390	**Urinary infection NOS (UTI)**
-	**Urinary tract lower, symptoms SEE LUTS**
N139	**Urinary tract obstruction NOS**
R339	**Urine retention NOS**
	drug induced R330
	other R338 psychogenic F458
	Possible RELATED code: enlarged prostate N401
N814	**Uterovaginal prolapse NOS**
	complete N813
	incomplete N812
N719	**Uterus abscess NOS**
	acute/subacute N710
	chronic N711
Z90710	**Uterus absence with cervix absence acquired**
	w/ remaining cervical stump acquired Z90711
N856	**Uterus adhesions/ bands internal**
N859	**Uterus disorders NOS**
	includes ulcer / fibrosis NOS / cyst / atrophy acquired
N800	**Uterus endometriosis**
N828	**Uterus fistula unsp**
N855	**Uterus inversion**
M854	**Uterus malposition / retroversion**

-	**Uterus neoplasm**
	MALIGNANT primary
	isthmus C540 endometrium C541
	myometrium C542 fundus uteri C543
	overlapping sites C548
	corpus uteri unsp C549
	Uterus NOS C55
	Secondary C7982
	Benign D261
	Mets to bone C7951 mets to unsp lymph nodes C779
	Mets to intrapelvic lymph node C775
N840	**Uterus polyp NOS**
N814	**Uterus prolapse NOS**
	with vagina prolapse -- SEE uterovaginal prolapse
N853	**Uterus subinvolution chronic**
N390	**UTI: urinary tract infection NOS**
N139	**UTO: urinary tract obstruction NOS**
T880XX-	**Vaccination infected**
	7th character indicates encounter
	A - initial encounter D - subsequent encounter S - sequela
Q872	**VACTERL: vertebrae anus cardiac trachea esophagus renal limbs**
Z452	**VAD: vascular access device - adjustment & management**
N895	**Vagina adhesions / atresia NOS**
	postop N992
B373	**Vagina candidiasis/moniliasis**
	aka VAGINAL THRUSH, yeast infection
S3023x-	**Vagina contusion**
	7th character indicates encounter
	A - initial encounter D - subsequent encounter S - sequela
N898	**Vagina cyst NOS**
	incl: of wall / inclusion / squamous cell
N898	**Vagina discharge/leukorrhea NOS**
N899	**Vagina disorder unsp noninflammatory**
N893	**Vagina dysplasia NOS SEE VAIN for intraepithelial neoplasia**
N804	**Vagina endometriosis**
N815	**Vagina enterocele NOS**
N829	**Vagina fistula NOS**
	to small intestine N822 to large intestine N823
	to skin / abdominal wall N825
	to bladder N820 other urinary tract N821
	other intetinal tract N824
	other N828
N898	**Vagina hematoma NOS / hemorrhage NOS**
A6004	**Vagina herpes simplex**
R87623	**Vagina high grade squamous intraepithelial lesion from pap smear**
A5602	**Vagina infection d/t chlamydia trachomatis**
B373	**Vagina infection yeast (candidiasis)**
N898	**Vagina laceration old (includes postop)**
N894	**Vagina leukoplakia**

N7681	**Vagina mucositis ulcerative**
	RELATED radiotherapy Y842
	RELATED antineoplastic drug poisoning
	-- accidental T451X1- adverse effect T451X5-
	-- undetermined T451X4-
	For T codes 7th character indicates encounter
	A - initial encounter D - subsequent encounter S - sequela
-	**Vagina neoplasm**
	Malignant primary C52
	Secondary C7982
	Benign D281
	Mets to bone C7951 mets to unsp lymph nodes C779
	Mets to intraabdominal lymph node C772
	Mets to intrapelvic lymph node C775
N842	**Vagina polyp**
N8189	**Vagina prolapse NOS w/o uterine prolapse**
	of vault after hysterectomy N993
	with uterus prolapse -- SEE uterovaginal prolapse
	Vagina posterior wall prolapse N816
	anterior wall: NOS N8110 midline N8111 lateral N8112
N895	**Vagina stricture / stenosis**
	also atresia
N942	**Vaginismus**
	functional/psychogenic F525
N760	**Vaginitis acute / NOS**
	chronic / subacute N761
	postmenopausal atrophic N952
	trichomonal A5901
	in other diseases N771
	RELATED pinworm B80
N890	**VAIN: vaginal intraepithelial neoplasia mild grade I**
	moderate grade II N891
	severe grade III D072
-	**Varicella SEE Chickenpox**
I8390	**Varicose veins NOS asymptomatic**
	scrotum I861 sublingual I860
	pelvis I862 vulva I863
	gastric I864
	other sites specified NEC I868
	SEE leg varicose veins and Esophagus varices
Z452	**Vascular access device adjustment and management**
R55	**Vasovagal attack**
Q872	**VATER: vertebrae anus trachea esophagus renal**
I871	**VCS: vena cava syndrome**
M5382	**VDTS: video display tube syndrome**
R403	**Vegetative state persistent**

-		**Venous central catheter infection**
		bloodstream infection T80211-
		local T80212-
		other T80218-
		unsp T80219-
		7th character indicates encounter
		A - initial encounter D - subsequent encounter S - sequela
K432		**Ventral hernia incisional NOS**
		incarcerated K430
		gangrenous K431
M4850x-		**Vertebrae collapsed / wedged unsp**
		occipito-atlanto-axial M4851x-
		cervical M4852x-
		cervicothoracic M4853x-
		thoracic M4854x- lumbar M4856x-
		thoracolumbar M4855x-
		lumbosacral M4857x-
		sacral and sacrococcygeal M4858x-
		7th character indicates encounter:
		A = initial encounter D = subsequent encounter, routine healing
		G = subsequent encounter, delayed healing S = sequela
M4840x-		**Vertebrae fracture fatigue unsp**
		occipito-atlanto-axial M4841x-
		cervical M4842x-
		cervicothoracic M4843x-
		thoracic M4844x- lumbar M4846x-
		thoracolumbar M4845x-
		lumbosacral M4847x-
		sacral and sacrococcygeal M4848x-
		7th character indicates encounter:
		A = initial encounter D = subsequent encounter, routine healing
		G = subsequent encounter, delayed healing S = sequela
-		**Vertebrae gout acute/NOS**
		idiopathic/primary M1008
		lead induced M1018
		drug induced M1028
		d/t renal impairment M1038
		other secondary M1048
-		**Vertebrae gout chronic**
		idiopathic/primary M1A08x-
		lead induced M1A18x-
		drug induced M1A28x-
		d/t renal impairment M1A38x-
		other secondary M1A48x-
		The appropriate 7th character
		0 = without tophus (tophi) 1 = with tophus (tophi)
M2508		**Vertebrae hemarthrosis**

M8008x-	**Vertebrae osteoporosis age related w/current pathological fracture**
	7th character indicates encounter/status
	A - initial S - sequela
	D - subsequent routine healing
	G - subsequent delayed healing
	K - subsequent nonunion P - subsequent malunion
-	**Vertebral artery compression syndromes**
	unsp site: M47029
	cervical: M47022
	occipito-atlanto-axial: M47021
I7774	**Vertebral artery dissection**
I6509	**Vertebral artery unsp occlusion / stenosis NOS**
	right I6501 left I6502
	bilat I6403
H8190	**Vertigo (vertiginous) syndrome NOS**
	right ear H8191 left ear H8192
	bilateral H8193
H8110	**Vertigo benign positional paroxysmal vertigo NOS**
	right ear H8111 left ear H8112
	bilateral H8113
H8109	**Vertigo Meniere's NOS**
	right ear H8101 left ear H8102
	bilateral H8103
	AKA: Meniere's syndrome; labyrinthine hydrops
R42	**Vertigo NOS**
-	**Vertigo otogenic SEE vertigo peripheral NOS**
H81399	**Vertigo peripheral NOS**
	right ear H81391 left ear H81392
	bilateral H81393
	AKA otogenic vertigo; Lemoyez' syndrome
N322	**Vesical fistula NEC (excludes fistula to female genital tract)**
R301	**Vesical tenesmus**
N321	**Vesicointestinal fistula**
N1370	**Vesicoureteral reflux unsp**
	specified w/o reflux nephropathy N1371
-	**Vesicoureteral reflux w/reflux nephropathy**
	unilateral N13721 w/hydroureter N13731
	bilateral: N13722 w/hydroureter N13732
	unspec: N13729 w/hydroureter N13739
N820	**Vesicovaginal fistula**
	other female urinary-genital fistulae N821
N900	**VIN: vulvar intraepithelial neoplasia type I mild**
	type II N901 type III/severe D071
B349	**Viremia**
	viral infection NOS
-	**Vitamin deficiency SEE Deficiency (vitamin)**

H4310	**Vitreous hemorrhage unsp** right eye H4311 left eye H4312 bilateral H4313
E781	**VLDL: very low density lipoid hyperlipoproteinemia**
R825	**VMA: vanillylmandelic acid elevated in urine**
T796XX-	**Volkmann's contractures ischemic** 7th character indicates encounter A - initial encounter D - subsequent encounter S - sequela
R1110	**Vomiting NOS** w/o nausea R1111 w/nausea unsp R112 projectile R1112 bilious R1114 fecal matter R1113 hematemesis K920 post-op GI surgery K910 cyclical: G43A0 intractable w/migraine G43A1
E7401	**von Gierke disease**
Z1621	**VRE: vancomycin resistant enterococcus (first code infection)**
Z1621	**VRSA: vancomycin resistant staph aureus (first code infection)**
Q210	**VSD: ventricular septal defect congenital**
N764	**Vulva abscess / furuncle**
N905	**Vulva atrophy** also stenosis
B373	**Vulva candidiasis/moniliasis**
N907	**Vulva cyst**
N909	**Vulva disorder unsp noninflammatory**
N903	**Vulva dysplasia other than VIN** SEE VIN for intraepithelial dysplasia
D071	**Vulva dysplasia severe**
N904	**Vulva dystrophy / kraurosis / leukoplakia**
N808	**Vulva endometriosis**
N9089	**Vulva hematoma**
N906	**Vulva hypertrophy NOS**
A5602	**Vulva infection d/t chlamydia trachomatis**
N9089	**Vulva laceration old /scarring**
N7681	**Vulva mucositis ulcerative** RELATED radiotherapy Y842 RELATED antineoplastic drug poisoning accidental T45.1X1- adverse effect T45.1X5- undetermined T45.1X4- For T codes 7th character indicates encounter A - initial encounter D - subsequent encounter S - sequela

-	**Vulva neoplasm**
	MALIGNANT primary
	labium majus C510 labium minus C511
	clitoris C512 overlapping sites C518
	unsp / NOS C519
	Secondary C7982
	Benign D280
	Mets to bone C7951 mets to unsp lymph nodes C779
	Mets to intraabdominal lymph node C772
	Mets to intrapelvic lymph node C775
N843	**Vulva polyp**
N9089	**Vulva stricture**
N766	**Vulva ulcer NOS**
	in gonococcal infection A5402
	in herpesviral [herpes simplex] infection A6004
	in syphilis A510
	in tuberculosis A1818
	in other diseases classified elsewhere N770
A6004	**Vulva ulceration herpetic**
I863	**Vulva varices**
N94810	**Vulva vestibulitis**
N942	**Vulvismus**
N762	**Vulvitis NOS or acute**
	subacute / chronic N763
N94819	**Vulvodynia NOS**
	Vulvodynia vestibulitis N94810
	other N94818
N751	**Vulvovaginal gland abscess**
N760	**Vulvovaginitis NOS / acute**
	subacute / chronic N761
	candidal/monilial B373
	gonococcal A5402 trichomonal B5809
	herpetic (simplex) A6004
	in other diseases N771
B373	**VVC: vulvovaginal candidiasis**
R262	**Walking difficulty NOS**
	ataxic gait R260 paralytic gait R261
	unsteady on feet R2681 other spec R2689
	unspecified gait difficulty R269
I498	**WAP: wandering atrial pacemaker**
B079	**Warts viral unspecified**
	common B078
	plantar B070
E41	**Wasting d/t malnutrition NOS / extreme**
G1221	**Wasting d/t paralysis (muscle atrophy)**
R64	**Wasting disease / syndrome - Code underlying condition first if known**

M6250	**Wasting of muscles NOS (disuse atrophy NEC)**
	shoulder: right M62511 left M62512 unsp M62519
	upper arm: right M62521 left M62522 unsp M62529
	forearm: right M62531 left M62532 unsp M62539
	hand: right M62541 left M62542 unsp M62549
	thigh: right M62551 left M62552 unsp M62559
	lower leg: right M62561 left M62562 unsp M62569
	ankle & foot: right M62571 left M62572 unsp M62579
	other site M6258
	multiple sites NEC M6259
D72829	**WBC count high NOS**
	lymphocytosis D72820 monocytosis D72821
	Plasmacytosis D72822 leukemoid reactiion D72823
	Basophilia D72824 Bandemia D72825 other D72828
D72819	**WBC count low NOS**
	lymphocytopenia D72810
	other D72818
R531	**Weakness NOS**
	age related R54
A831	**WEE: Western equine encephalitis**
M3130	**Wegener's granulomatosis/syndrome**
	w/renal involvement M3131
R636	**Weight below normal (Code body mass index if known)**
R635	**Weight gain abnormal**
R634	**Weight loss abnormal**
E512	**Wernicke's encephalopathy / syndrome**
A9230	**West Nile Fever NOS**
	w/encephalitis A9231
	w/neuro complication except encephalitis A9232
	w/complication other than neuro A9239
Z993	**Wheelchair dependence**
	Code cause first
Z4689	**Wheelchair fitting & adjustment**
R062	**Wheezing**
	do not code with asthma
A9230	**WNF: West Nile Fever NOS**
	w/encephalitis A9231
	w/other neuro manifestations A9232
	w/other complications A9239
A4852	**Wound botulism**
-	**Wound care**
	change/remove dsg nonsurgica/NOS wound Z4800
	change/remove dsg surgical wound Z4801
	remove sutures or staples Z4802
	change/remove drain Z4803

	Wound dehiscence
	wound disruption NOS T8130x-
	surgical wound skin & subcut tissue disruption T8131x-
	surgical wound deep / internal disruption T8132x-
	of traumatic injury wound repair T8133x-
	For above codes, 7th character indicates encounter
	A - initial encounter D - subsequent encounter S - sequela
	of amputation stump T8781
Z4803	**Wound drain postop change / removal**
T814xx-	**Wound infection postop NEC any site except OB**
	7th character indicates encounter
	A - initial encounter D - subsequent encounter S - sequela
	Use additional code to identify infection
T8189X-	**Wound surgical non-healing**
	7th character indicates encounter
	A - initial encounter D - subsequent encounter S - sequela
I456	**WPW: Wolff Parkinson White syndrome**
M25739	**Wrist bone spur (osteophyte) unsp**
	right M25731 left M25732
M71439	**Wrist calcification unsp**
	right M71431 left M71432
M94239	**Wrist chondromalacia unsp**
	right M94231 left M94232
M21339	**Wrist drop acquired unsp**
	right M21331 left M21332
-	**Wrist gout acute/NOS**
	idiopathic/primary right M10031 left M10032 unsp M10039
	lead induced right M10131 left M10132 unsp M10139
	drug induced right M10231 left M10232 unsp M10239
	d/t renal impairment right M10331 left M10332 unsp M10339
	other secondary right M10431 left M10432 unsp M10439
-	**Wrist gout chronic**
	idiopathic/primary right M1A031- left M1A032- unsp M1A039-
	lead induced right M1A131- left M1A132- unsp M1A139-
	drug induced right M1A231- left M1A232- unsp M1A239-
	d/t renal impairment right M1A331- left M1A332- unsp M1A339-
	other secondary right M1A431- left M1A432- unsp M1A439-
	The appropriate 7th character
	0 = without tophus (tophi) 1 = with tophus (tophi)
M25039	**Wrist hemarthrosis unsp**
	right M25031 left M25032
M25539	**Wrist pain unsp**
	right M25531 left M25532
R238	**Xanthosis**
-	**Zona - SEE Herpes Zoster**

Made in the USA
Lexington, KY
24 August 2015